Novel Therapies in Hepatitis C Virus

Guest Editor

PAUL J. POCKROS, MD

CLINICS IN LIVER DISEASE

www.liver.theclinics.com

Consulting Editor
NORMAN GITLIN, MD

August 2009 • Volume 13 • Number 3

SAUNDERS an imprint of ELSEVIER, Inc.

W.B. SAUNDERS COMPANY

A Division of Elsevier Inc.

1600 John F. Kennedy Boulevard, Suite 1800 • Philadelphia, PA 19103-2899

http://www.theclinics.com

CLINICS IN LIVER DISEASE Volume 13, Number 3
August 2009 ISSN 1089-3261, ISBN-13: 978-1-4377-1236-0, ISBN-10: 1-4377-1236-3

Editor: Kerry Holland
Developmental Editor: Donald Mumford

Clinics in Liver Disease (ISSN 1089-3261) is published quarterly by Elsevier Inc., 360 Park Avenue South, New York, NY 10010-1710. Months of issue are February, May, August, and November. Business and editorial offices: 1600 John F. Kennedy Boulevard, Suite 1800, Philadelphia, PA 19103-2899. Customer service office: 6277 Sea Harbor Drive, Orlando, FL 32887-4800. Periodicals postage paid at New York, NY, and additional mailing offices. Subscription prices are $218.00 per year (U.S. individuals), $109.00 per year (U.S. student/resident), $333.00 per year (U.S. institutions), $288.00 per year (foreign individuals), $151.00 per year (foreign student/resident), $401.00 per year (foreign instituitions), $251.00 per year (Canadian individuals), $151.00 per year (Canadian student/resident), and $401.00 per year (Canadian institutions). Foreign air speed delivery is included in all *Clinics* subscription prices. All prices are subject to change without notice. **POSTMASTER:** Send address changes to *Clinics in Liver Disease*, Elsevier Journals Customer Service, 11830 Westline Industrial Drive, St. Louis, MO 63146. **Customer Service (orders, claims, online, change of address): Elsevier Periodicals Customer Service, 11830 Westline Industrial Drive, St. Louis, MO 63146. Tel: 1-800-654-2452 (U.S. and Canada); 314-453-7041 (outside U.S. and Canada). Fax: 314-453-5170. E-mail: journalscustomerservice-usa@elsevier.com (for print support); journalsonlinesupport-usa@elsevier.com (for online support).**

Reprints. For copies of 100 or more of articles in this publication, please contact the Commercial Reprints Department, Elsevier Inc., 360 Park Avenue South, New York, NY 10010-1710. Tel.: 212-633-3812; Fax: 212-462-1935; E-mail: reprints@elsevier.com.

Clinics in Liver Disease is covered in *MEDLINE/PubMed (Index Medicus).*

Printed and bound in the United Kingdom
Transferred to Digital Print 2011

Contributors

GUEST EDITOR

PAUL J. POCKROS, MD
Head, Division of Gastroenterology and Hepatology; Director, SC Liver Research Consortium, Scripps Clinic; Skaggs Scholar, The Scripps Research Institute, La Jolla, California

AUTHORS

KENNETH BERMAN, MD
Division of Gastroenterology and Hepatology, Indiana University School of Medicine, Indianapolis, Indiana

AYBIKE BIRERDINC, PhD
Research Project Associate, Betty and Guy Beatty Center for Integrated Research, Inova Health System, Falls Church, Virginia

JAMES R. BURTON, Jr., MD
Assistant Professor of Medicine, Medical Director of Liver Transplantation, Division of Gastroenterology and Hepatology, University of Colorado Denver, Aurora, Colorado

VIRGINIA CLARK, MD, MS
Assistant Professor, Division of Gastroenterology, Hepatology, and Nutrition, Department of Medicine, University of Florida, Gainesville, Florida

GEOFFREY DUSHEIKO, MB, BCh, FCP(SA), FRCP, FRCP(Edin)
Professor of Medicine, Centre for Hepatology, Royal Free and University College School of Medicine, Royal Free Hospital, Hampstead, London

GREGORY T. EVERSON, MD
Professor of Medicine and Director of Hepatology, Division of Gastroenterology and Hepatology, University of Colorado Denver, Aurora, Colorado

KIMBERLY A. FORDE, MD, MHS
Instructor, Division of Gastroenterology, Department of Medicine, University of Pennsylvania; Clinical Epidemiology and Biostatistics, School of Medicine, University of Pennsylvania, Philadelphia, Pennsylvania

PHILIPPE A. GALLAY, PhD
Associate Professor, Department of Immunology and Microbial Science, The Scripps Research Institute, California

GREGORY J. GORES, MD
Professor of Medicine, Division of Gastroenterology and Hepatology, Miles and Shirley Fiterman Center for Digestive Diseases, College of Medicine, Mayo Clinic, Rochester, Minnesota

MARIA EUGENIA GUICCIARDI, PhD
Assistant Professor of Medicine, Division of Gastroenterology and Hepatology, Miles and Shirley Fiterman Center for Digestive Diseases, College of Medicine, Mayo Clinic, Rochester, Minnesota

IRA M. JACOBSON, MD
Chief, Division of Gastroenterology and Hepatology, Department of Medicine; Vincent Astor Professor of Medicine, Weill Cornell Medical College, New York Presbyterian Hospital, New York

PAUL Y. KWO, MD
Associate Professor of Medicine and Medical Director of Liver Transplantation, Division of Gastroenterology and Hepatology, Indiana University School of Medicine, Indianapolis, Indiana

HOWARD C. MASUOKA, MD, PhD
Instructor of Medicine, Division of Gastroenterology and Hepatology, Miles and Shirley Fiterman Center for Digestive Diseases, College of Medicine, Mayo Clinic, Rochester, Minnesota

HESHAAM M. MIR, MD
Clinical Researcher, Center for Liver Diseases, Inova Fairfax Hospital; Betty and Guy Beatty Center for Integrated Research, Inova Health System, Falls Church, Virginia

DAVID R. NELSON, MD
Professor, Division of Gastroenterology, Hepatology and Nutrition, Department of Medicine; Medical Director of Liver Transplantation Program, University of Florida, Gainesville, Florida

KEYUR PATEL, MD
Assistant Professor of Medicine, Division of Gastroenterology and Hepatology, Duke Clinical Research Institute, Duke University, Durham, North Carolina

PAUL J. POCKROS, MD
Head, Division of Gastroenterology and Hepatology; Director, SC Liver Research Consortium, Scripps Clinic; Skaggs Scholar, The Scripps Research Institute, La Jolla, California

K. RAJENDER REDDY, MD
Professor of Medicine and Medical Director of Liver Transplantation, Division of Gastroenterology, Department of Medicine, University of Pennsylvania, Philadelphia, Pennsylvania

WILLIAM W. SHIELDS, DO
Department of Gastroenterology and Hepatology, Naval Medical Center San Diego, San Diego, California

ALEXANDER J.V. THOMPSON, MD, PhD
Clinical Research Fellow, Division of Gastroenterology and Hepatology, Duke Clinical Research Institute, Duke University, Durham, North Carolina

ILAN S. WEISBERG, MD, MSc
Clinical Fellow, Division of Gastroenterology and Hepatology, Center for the Study of Hepatitis C, Department of Medicine, Weill Cornell Medical College, New York Presbyterian Hospital, New York

ZOBAIR M. YOUNOSSI, MD, MPH
Executive Director of Research, Betty and Guy Beatty Center for Integrated Research, Inova Health System; Executive Director, Center for Liver Diseases, Inova Fairfax Hospital, Falls Church, Virginia

Contents

Preface **xiii**

Paul J. Pockros

Novel Interferons for Treatment of Hepatitis C Virus **351**

Virginia Clark and David R. Nelson

The current standard of care for treatment of hepatitis C is pegylated interferon and ribavirin. Despite the large number of new oral agents under development, interferon will likely remain the backbone of future therapy. Interferon has unique antiviral and immunomodulatory properties, which have been critical in limiting resistance to protease inhibitors and improving efficacy. Hence, optimizing pharmacokinetics and promoting adherence to interferon dosing regimens will become even more critical as new regimens enter the clinical arena. This review highlights novel interferons under development that may offer therapeutic advantages over the formulations currently available.

Antifibrotics for Chronic Hepatitis C **365**

Paul J. Pockros

Development and testing of antifibrotic agents for the treatment of chronic hepatitis C have generally been targeted toward hepatic stellate cells, transforming growth factor-β, the inflammatory response, or extracellular matrix accumulation. Although several agents such as interferon-γ, long-term pegylated interferon, and caspase inhibitors have been studied, none have proved to be effective to date. There is a clear need for drugs that inhibit or reverse hepatic fibrosis as these would be immediately applicable to patients for whom antiviral therapy has failed or who have contraindications to antiviral therapy such as those with decompensated liver disease or renal failure. A major impediment in the development of new drugs in this field has been the inability to identify appropriate histologic or clinical end points within a reasonable period of study. Progress on providing suitable end points to therapy will then promote the development of newer agents.

Antisense Inhibitors, Ribozymes, and siRNAs **375**

Alexander J.V. Thompson and Keyur Patel

The current standard of care for the treatment of hepatitis C virus infection, pegylated interferon-α and ribavirin, is costly, associated with significant side effects, and effective in only 50% of patients. There is therefore a need for the development of novel antiviral therapies. One such approach involves the application of gene silencing technologies, including antisense oligonucleotides, ribozymes, RNA interference, and aptamers. However, despite great scientific advances over the past decade, and promising in vitro data, several significant challenges continue to limit the translation of this technology to the clinical setting. This review provides a concise update of the current literature.

Hepatitis C Virus Infection and Immunomodulatory Therapies **391**

Kimberly A. Forde and K. Rajender Reddy

Hepatitis C virus (HCV) infection remains a large-scale and significant health concern. The combination of subcutaneously administered pegylated interferon and oral ribavirin is the FDA-approved regimen for the treatment of chronic HCV infection. Combination therapy may result in a sustained virologic response leading to HCV eradication, with a reduction in risk for cirrhosis, hepatic decompensation, and hepatocellular carcinoma.9,10 However, the combination of PEG-IFN and ribavirin does not universally result in cure in all patients who undergo treatment. In this article, the authors discuss immunomodulatory therapies and clinical trials in the treatment of HCV infection.

Cyclophilin Inhibitors **403**

Philippe A. Gallay

The percentage of patients chronically infected with hepatitis C virus (HCV) who have reached sustained antiviral response has increased since the introduction of the pegylated interferon-alpha (pIFNa) and ribavirin (RBV) treatment. However, the current standard pIFNa/RBV therapy not only has a low success rate (about 50%) but is often associated with serious side effects. Thus, there is an urgent need for the development of new anti-HCV agents. Cyclophilin (Cyp) inhibitors are among the most promising of the new anti-HCV agents under development. Recent clinical studies demonstrate that Cyp inhibitors are potent anti-HCV drugs, with a novel mechanism of action and efficacy profiles that make them attractive candidates for combination with current and future HCV treatments.

Ribavirin Analogs **419**

William W. Shields and Paul J. Pockros

Ribavirin is ineffective against hepatitis C virus as mono-therapy but is critical in attaining both early virologic response and sustained virologic response when combined with pegylated interferon. Ribavirin has significant dose-limiting toxicities, the most important of which is hemolytic anemia. Taribavirin is a ribavirin pro-drug, which targets the liver and has less incidence of anemia, and it may be a promising alternative to ribavirin in the future.

Boceprevir, an NS3 Protease Inhibitor of HCV **429**

Kenneth Berman and Paul Y. Kwo

Hepatitis C virus (HCV) is a major cause of chronic liver disease leading to death from liver failure or hepatocellular carcinoma. Hepatitis C is the most common indication for liver transplantation worldwide and is a major cause of the increased incidence of hepatocellular cancer in the United States. The current paradigm for HCV treatment relies on pegylated interferon and ribavirin as agents that enhance endogenous mechanisms for viral clearance and are dependent on host factors. In patients with genotype 1 HCV infection, sustained viral response (SVR) rates remain suboptimal, with less than half of genotype 1–infected individuals going on to achieve SVR. This has led to a shift in the investigational focus for treatment of HCV toward specifically targeted antiviral therapy for HCV agents. This review focuses on boceprevir, a protease inhibitor, and discusses its mechanism of action, effects on HCV, and viral resistance.

Telaprevir: Hope on the Horizon, Getting Closer **441**

Ilan S. Weisberg and Ira M. Jacobson

Standard therapy with pegylated interferon and ribavirin for chronic hepatitis C is effective in 40% to 50% of individuals with genotype 1 hepatitis C virus (HCV) infection and is associated with significant treatment-related toxicities. Newly developed small molecules that target key enzymes essential for HCV replication are in development. Telaprevir, a peptidomimetic inhibitor of the HCV NS3/4A protease, has shown great promise in early trials and is currently in advanced stages of clinical development. In treatment-naïve patients and those with previous treatment failure, the addition of telaprevir to standard interferon and ribavirin therapy is well tolerated and enhances rates of sustained virologic response while shortening the treatment duration. In this report, the current experience using telaprevir to treat chronic HCV infection as monotherapy and in combination with other agents is reviewed.

HCV NS5B Polymerase Inhibitors **453**

James R. Burton, Jr. and Gregory T. Everson

Chronic hepatitis C virus (HCV) infection affects approximately 4 million persons and is the major indication for liver transplantation in the United States. The current standard for treatment of HCV is pegylated interferon in combination with ribavirin. Despite significant advances in treatment, only approximately 50% of patients of treated patients clear HCV infection. Polymerase inhibitors, given their potent antiviral effects, represent a major contribution to the future of HCV treatment. Whether these new drugs will have a role in the treatment of the difficult patient (non-responders, those co-infected with HIV, decompensated liver disease and liver transplant recipients) remains to be determined.

Caspase Inhibitors for the Treatment of Hepatitis C **467**

Howard C. Masuoka, Maria Eugenia Guicciardi, and Gregory J. Gores

Decreasing hepatocyte injury and death is an attractive therapeutic target in chronic hepatitis C and other liver diseases. Apoptotic cell death is a critical mechanism responsible for liver injury in hepatitis C, and contributes to hepatic fibrogenesis. At the cellular level, apoptosis is executed by a family of cysteine proteases termed caspases. Caspase inhibitors have been developed to inhibit these proteases and attenuate cellular apoptosis in vivo. By reducing hepatocyte apoptosis these agents have the potential to serve as hepatoprotective agents, minimizing liver injury and fibrosis. Studies on a variety of animal models, and time-limited studies in human patients with hepatitis C suggest these are promising therapeutic agents. However, although these agents hold promise, their usefulness requires further studies, especially longer duration studies using hepatic fibrogenesis as the end point before they can be considered further for the treatment of patients infected with the hepatitis C virus.

Monoclonal and Polyclonal Antibodies Against the HCV Envelope Proteins **477**

Heshaam M. Mir, Aybike Birerdinc, and Zobair M. Younossi

The potential for developing efficient and efficacious therapies for hepatitis C virus continues to improve. Insight into the molecular processes involved in attachment, entry, and fusion suggests that antibodies could potentially inhibit viral replication at any or all of these stages, and the attachment and entry stages present the best target for antibodies that can attack the virus. Monoclonal and polyclonal antibodies present an important therapeutic option in this area, and this article assesses current investigations of several antibodies.

Thrombopoietin Agonists for the Treatment of Thrombocytopenia in Liver Disease and Hepatitis C **487**

Geoffrey Dusheiko

Thrombocytopenia is a condition of unusually low level of platelets in blood, resulting from an imbalance between the production and destruction of platelets, and is associated with aplastic anemia, myelodysplasia, and idiopathic thrombocytopenic purpura (ITP). Thrombocytopenia can also be associated with severe chronic liver disease as a result of several factors that may act in concert, including reduced production of the endogenous thrombopoietic growth factor, thrombopoietin (TPO). This article examines the nature of thrombocytopenia, ITP, and TPO.

Index **503**

FORTHCOMING ISSUES

November 2009
Non-Alcoholic Steatohepatitis
Stephen A. Harrison, MD, *Guest Editor*

February 2010
Liver Disease and Endoscopy
Andres Cardenas, MD, and
Paul J. Thuluvath, MD, *Guest Editors*

May 2010
Healthcare-Associated Viral Hepatitis
Bandar Al Knawy, MD, FRCPC,
Guest Editor

RECENT ISSUES

May 2009
Key Consultations in Hepatology
Paul Martin, MD, *Guest Editor*

February 2009
Coagulation and Hemostasis in Liver Disease: Controversies and Advances
Stephen H. Caldwell, MD, and
Arun J. Sanyal, MD, *Guest Editors*

November 2008
Hepatic Fibrosis: Pathogenesis, Diagnosis, and Emerging Therapies
Scott L. Friedman, MD, *Guest Editor*

RELATED INTEREST

Infectious Disease Clinics of North America, March 2006, Vol. 20, No. 1
Hepatitis
R.C. Moellering, Jr., *Guest Editor*

Preface

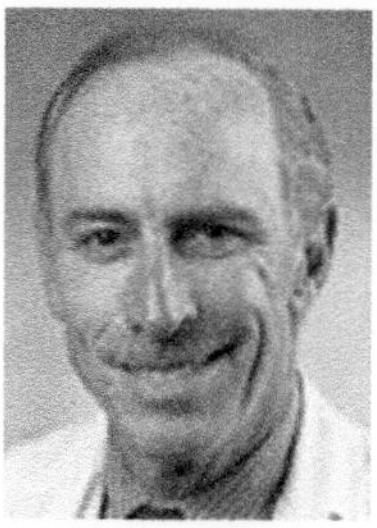

Paul J. Pockros, MD
Guest Editor

The current standard of care for chronic hepatitis C therapy is a combination of pegylated interferon and ribavirin. Eradication of the hepatitis C virus (HCV) has been proved to be possible in roughly half of all patients treated; however, viral eradication rates are superior in patients with viral genotypes 2 and 3 compared with genotype 1 patients.

Current therapies have significant adverse events besides a less-than-ideal sustained virologic response in genotype 1 patients. For this reason, it is imperative that we have new drugs for treatment of HCV, particularly genotype 1 disease. The novel agents discussed herein will become a crucial part of treatment regimens for HCV as soon as they become available. Furthermore, many treating physicians and patients are waiting for these new classes of agents and deferring current therapy. The promise of improved efficacy and shorter duration of therapy is a beacon for the future. These drugs are essentially in a race for approval, against each other and against the huge tide of HCV-infected individuals who have had the disease for 30 years or more. Many of these patients are facing advanced disease, complications or cirrhosis, hepatocellular carcinoma, and death or transplant if their disease is not eradicated.

This issue of *Clinics in Liver Disease* has articles written by top experts; it serves as a compilation that comprehensively reviews these novel therapies and that should prepare hepatologists as these regimens become available.

Paul J. Pockros, MD
Division of Gastroenterology and Hepatology
The Scripps Research Institute
10666 North Torrey Pines Road
La Jolla, CA 92037, USA

E-mail address:
pockros.paul@scrippshealth.org (P.J. Pockros)

Clin Liver Dis 13 (2009) xiii
doi:10.1016/j.cld.2009.06.001

Novel Interferons for Treatment of Hepatitis C Virus

Virginia Clark, MD, MS, David R. Nelson, MD*

KEYWORDS

- Hepatitis C • Interferon • Treatment • Antiviral
- Immunomodulatory

Since the discovery of interferon (IFN) more than 50 years ago, clinical uses have expanded across many disciplines of medicine.[1] Although IFN is the current backbone of treatment regimens for chronic hepatitis C (HCV), the initial choice of IFN for chronic non-A, non-B hepatitis was largely empiric, highly intuitive, and as is the case in many great scientific discoveries, a little bit lucky.[2,3] At the time of the first clinical trial, HCV had not been identified, and virologic testing was not even possible. Over the ensuing 20 years, a dramatic evolution in the use of IFN to treat chronic HCV has occurred.

The goal of treatment of HCV is a sustained virologic response (SVR), which is defined as undetectable levels of HCV RNA 24 weeks after completion of treatment. Initial studies with IFN as a single agent for the treatment of HCV demonstrated limited success, with SVR rates of 6% to 12% after 6 months of treatment.[4] By extending treatment to 48 weeks as recommended by the NIH Consensus Development Conference (standard IFN-α 3 million units 3 times a week), SVR rates improved to 16% to 20%.[4,5] The next step forward for HCV therapy was the addition of ribavirin (RBV) to standard IFN, which improved SVR rates to 38% to 43% with 48 weeks of therapy.[6,7] Although the basic components of "combination therapy" have remained the same over the last decade, much effort has been invested to determine the optimal delivery of the IFN and RBV components.

The pharmacokinetic characteristics of standard IFN-α are such that sustained plasma levels are not maintained when dosed 3 times weekly, which is believed in part to explain the suboptimal response rates.[8] Adding a polyethylene glycol (PEG) polymer to IFN-α2a/b successfully created a molecule with a longer half-life, improved pharmacokinetic profile, and more importantly, a superior clinical response when dosed once weekly.[9–11] Large, randomized, controlled trials with PEG-IFN-α2a/b in

Division of Gastroenterology, Hepatology, and Nutrition, Department of Medicine, University of Florida, 1600 SW Archer Rd, Room M440, PO Box 100214, Gainesville, FL 32610, USA
* Corresponding author.
E-mail address: nelsodr@medicine.ufl.edu (D.R. Nelson).

Clin Liver Dis 13 (2009) 351–363
doi:10.1016/j.cld.2009.05.004
1089-3261/09/$ – see front matter

combination with ribavirin demonstrated overall SVR rates of 54% to 56%, which has now been established as the current standard of care for chronic HCV.[12–14] The safety of PEG-IFN-α is well established, and the side effect profile is well known. The current formulations of PEG-IFN have similar side effect profiles, including fatigue, headache, fever, myalgias, insomnia, alopecia, irritability, dermatitis, injection site reactions, and depression.[15] As many as 10% of patients may discontinue treatment because of side effects, and 32% to 42% may have dose reductions related to cytopenias.[12,13] A wealth of clinical experience has led to therapeutic strategies to manage adverse events and the impact they have on quality of life, but an opportunity exists to improve on the IFNs that are currently available.[16,17] These substantial gains made since the days of IFN-α monotherapy are encouraging; however, approximately half of the patients with HCV are not cured with the current therapy, and many others are not able to tolerate these regimens, underscoring the importance of the development of new drugs.

Much of the current effort in new therapies for HCV is targeted at direct antiviral agents (STAT-C).[18,19] Several agents look promising, although a major concern is the emergence of a drug resistant virus once HCV is under strong selective pressure.[20] This is because HCV replication occurs at a high rate and with low accuracy, and if an antiviral agent is going to be successful as a single agent, it will need to have a high barrier to resistance. Until such an ideal antiviral molecule (or combination) exists, it is likely that any new agent will first be incorporated into the current standard of care for HCV.[21] Early data from the Telaprevir (a protease inhibitor) trials suggest that virologic breakthrough is associated with lower serum trough levels of protease inhibitor and/or PEG-IFN.[22] As the backbone of treatment, IFN-α can supply sustained antiviral pressure that can limit resistance. IFN-α also has potent antiviral activity and immunomodulatory properties that are important in achieving an SVR.[23] Hence, optimizing pharmacokinetics and promoting adherence to IFN dosing regimens will become even more critical as STAT-C regimens enter the clinical arena.

NEW INTERFERON-α MOLECULES

Each of the new IFNs under development offer a therapeutic advantage over the current standard of care (PEG-IFN). In theory, these new drugs would have some combination of (1) improved viral suppression, (2) more convenient dosing schedules, (3) optimized pharmacokinetic profiles or (4) reduced side effects. The ultimate result of any of these advancements must translate to improved SVR rates. A summary of each new IFN highlighted in this review is shown in **Table 1**.

Albumin-interferon

Albumin-interferon α2b (Alb-IFN) is the most mature of the newest generation of interferons as phase III trials are now being completed. Alb-IFN is an 85.7-kDa protein consisting of recombinant human IFN-α2b genetically fused to recombinant human albumin. The albumin-fusion platform is another approach to enhance the pharmacokinetics of IFN. Albumin has several features that make it an excellent candidate for a drug delivery platform, including a long half-life (approx. 19 days), a wide volume of distribution, and minimal potential for immunogenicity.[24] The pharmacologic challenge is to maintain the functional antiviral activity of IFN in this setting. Preclinical in vitro data demonstrated that Alb-IFN can activate IFN-specific signal-transduction pathways.[24] In addition, in an HCV replicon system, Alb-IFN inhibited HCV replication at a comparable level to PEG-IFN-α2a, and at clinically relevant serum concentrations, antiviral activity was greater than any of the PEG-IFNs.[25] In vivo studies with

Table 1
Summary of interferons under development

Drug Type	Postulated Advantages Over PEG-IFN	Study
Novel interferons		
Albumin-IFN (Human Genome Sciences/Novartis)	Optimize drug exposure for improved efficacy, improved dosing schedule, fewer side effects	Phase III
Consensus IFN (Three Rivers Pharma)	—	Approved
Gene-shuffled interferon-α (Maxygen)	Select favorable properties of IFN while minimizing dose limiting effects	Phase I
Hyperglycosylated IFN (Alios BioPharma)	improved pharmacokinetics that avoids decrease in antiviral activity	Preclinical
Novel delivery systems		
Locteron(Octoplus, Biolex Therapeutics)	Increased dosing interval with fewer side effects	Phase II
IFN-α2bXL (Flamel Technologies)	Increased dosing interval with fewer side effects	Phase I
Other interferons		
IFN-β	Shorter treatment duration of 24 wk	—
IFN-ω (Intarcia Therapeutics)	Improved efficacy with fewer side effects	Phase I/II
IFN-γ	Improved immunomodulatory effects	Phase I
IFN-λ (Zymogenetics)	Limited hematopoietic and central nervous system side effects with similar antiviral activity	Phase I/II
TLR agonists		
IMO-2125 (Idera)	Improved immunomodulatory properties of innate immune response	Phase I
CpG-10101 (Coley Pharmaceuticals, Pfizer)	Improved immunomodulatory properties of innate immune response	Phase I
ANA 733 (Anadys)	Improved immunomodulatory properties of innate immune response	Phase I
CpG B & CpG C (Dynavax Technologies)	Improved immunomodulatory properties of innate immune response	Preclinical

cynomolgus monkeys given a single dose of Alb-IFN demonstrated a long half-life as Alb-IFN was detected more than 7 days after a single dose, and evidence of antiviral activity was still present.[26] These in vitro and in vivo studies supported the further clinical development of Alb-IFN.

An initial phase I/II trial of escalating doses (10–900 mcg) of Alb-IFN given as a single dose or as 2 injections 14 days apart established a favorable safety profile and a mean elimination half-life of approximately 6.6 days in a group of previous IFN nonresponders.[27] IFN specific gene induction and antiviral activity was demonstrated at day 28 in patients after a single dose of Alb-IFN.[27,28] A phase II, open-label, dose-ranging (200–1200 mcg) study showed dose-dependent levels of antiviral activity with the greatest levels of viral suppression at the 900 mcg and 1200 mcg doses.[29] At these higher doses, continued viral suppression was noted 28 days after the second injection, providing rationale for further studies with dosing intervals of 2 and 4 weeks.[29]

In a recent phase IIb, randomized, open-label study, 3 groups of treatment naive patients with chronic HCV were treated with Alb-IFN and ribavirin and compared with a control group treated with PEG-IFN-α2a and ribavirin.[30] The first group (n = 118) was dosed at 2-week intervals with 900 mcg. In this group, the overall SVR was 58.5 (95% CI 49–67.5), which was comparable to the control group SVR of 57.9%. In the higher-dosed cohorts (1200 mcg every 2 weeks and 1200 mcg every 4 weeks), there was not a significant change in the reported SVR (55.5% and 50.9%, respectively). Overall, the safety profile of Alb-IFN was comparable to that of the control group, with no new adverse events being reported. Notably, the monthly dosing interval was associated with minimal cytopenias and was clearly well tolerated. Cough and dyspnea were higher in the cohort on Alb-IFN 1200 mcg every 2 weeks, as well as the overall rate of discontinuation secondary to adverse events. Health-related quality of life scores were better at the 900 mcg every 2 weeks dose and fewer days of work were missed during the first 3 months of treatment.[30] Thus, this pivotal phase II study suggested that Alb-IFN may offer improved delivery and tolerability, while delivering similar efficacy. Alb-IFN has also been studied in a group of patients who had not previously responded to IFN-based therapy.[31] Patients were initially dosed every 2 weeks with 900, 1200, 1500, and 1800 mcg of Alb-IFN to evaluate the safety and efficacy over a range of doses. The rate of severe adverse events increased as the dose increased. The overall SVR rate was 17%, which is not a substantial improvement over previously reported rates for this hard to treat patient population.[31]

Phase III trials with dosing of 900 and 1200 mcg/wk every 2 weeks have now been completed in genotype 1 naive (ACHIEVE 1) and genotype 2/3 (ACHIEVE 2/3) patients with HCV. The preliminary release of the results shows that both studies met the primary end point of noninferiority, however there was no reported benefit in quality of life or adverse event profile noted with the use of Alb-IFN.[32,33] In ACHIEVE 1, 48.2% of patients in the group treated with 900 mcg Alb-IFN achieved SVR, compared with 47.3% in the 1200 mcg group and 51% in the PEG-IFN-α2a control group. In ACHIEVE 2/3, SVR rates were 84.8%, 79.8%, and 80% in the PEG-IFN-α2a, Alb-IFN 900, and Alb-IFN 1200 groups, respectively. Across the 2 phase III trials, the overall percentage of patients who had serious or adverse events, or discontinued due to an adverse event was comparable in all dose groups: 23.2% in patients randomized to receive 900 mcg Alb-IFN; 26% in patients randomized to receive 1200 mcg Alb-IFN, and 21.6% in patients receiving PEG-α2a. Given these early reports from phase III trials, Alb-IFN will likely obtain approval from the US Food and Drug Administration (FDA), however it is still unclear how it will fit into the future landscape of HCV therapy. In addition, the highly desirable 4-weekly dosing regimens are just now undergoing further phase II evaluation.

Consensus Interferon-α

IFN alphacon-1 is a synthetic type I IFN that was created by aligning the sequences of several IFN-α subtypes and using the most commonly observed amino acid in each position to generate a consensus molecule.[34] The in vitro antiviral activity of IFN alphacon-1 is substantially better than that reported for standard IFN-α, providing the rationale that superior SVR rates may be obtainable.[35,36] The initial phase III study compared IFN alphacon-1 to standard IFN-α2b, and the clinical efficacy appeared similar (SVR 12% versus 11%).[37] A recent single-center study has also showed no difference in SVR between patients treated with IFN alphacon-1/ribavirin and PEG-IFN-α2b/ribavirin(37% versus 41%, respectively).[38] Because IFN alphacon-1 requires 3 injections per week compared with the single weekly injection required for pegylated formulations of IFN-α2a/b, it has been a challenge to integrate this drug into routine clinical practice. Of interest, a pegylated version of IFN alphacon-1 has been developed with phase I data presented, but no further development of this compound seems to be underway.[39] The role of IFN alphacon-1 in clinical practice currently seems to be limited to select groups of patients who have failed previous therapy (select group of nonresponders and relapsers) and who had an adequate duration of therapy with PEG-IFN and RBV initially.[40,41]

Gene-shuffled Interferon-α

DNA shuffling is an in vitro method that can be used to generate candidate genes with desired therapeutic properties.[42] The technique involves fragmenting the targeted gene in multiple ways and allowing the fragments to recombine at homologous sequences. The process is repeated until a library of full-length novel genes is generated. The library is then screened for the desired properties. IFN-α is well suited for DNA shuffling technology because it belongs to a large family of wild-type IFN genes, each with a range of antiviral, immunomodulatory, and antiproliferative effects. Ideally, a recombinant interferon could be created with maximal antiviral and immunomodulatory effects while minimizing the antiproliferative effects that are dose limiting (neutropenia and thrombocytopenia). A library of clones has been generated (Maxygen) with the proof of concept demonstrated. Several clones have been identified through this process of directed evolution that have improved antiviral activity in vitro compared with IFN-α2b and IFN-α-con1.[43] One of these compounds (MAXY-alpha) was advanced to phase I development. However, preliminary observations (Hoffman-La Roche, press release, September 21, 2007, Nutley, NJ) from a phase I trial indicated that an unexpected reduction of the pharmacodynamic and pharmacokinetic effects of MAXY-alpha occurred in most subjects who received 2 doses. In addition, antibodies binding to MAXY-alpha were identified in some subjects. The sponsor has initiated additional investigational studies to assess these results and further clinical development seems to be on hold.

Hyperglycosylated IFN

Post-transcriptional modification with carbohydrate moieties can successfully increase the molecular weight and improve the pharmacokinetic characteristics of therapeutic proteins.[44] Hyperglycosylation of IFN could provide an alternate mechanism for improved pharmacokinetics that may avoid the in vitro decrease in specific antiviral activity that occurs after pegylation for PEG-IFN-α2a and PEG-IFN-α2b.[45,46] A consensus IFN with the primary amino acid sequence modified to encode for additional glycosylation sites has been developed (Alios BioPharma).[47] Preclinical data suggest this might be a viable strategy and further clinical development is anticipated.[47]

NOVEL DELIVERY SYSTEMS FOR INTERFERON-α

The advantage PEG- IFN offered over standard IFN was maintenance of adequate drug levels and antiviral activity at decreased dosing intervals. Alternatively, novel delivery systems are being developed that use methods for controlled release of unmodified IFN-α to achieve sustained therapeutic levels. One such drug is Locteron (Octoplus, Biolex Therapeutics), which is recombinant IFN-α2b synthesized in a *Lemna* aquatic plant expression system, and embedded in biodegradable poly(ether-ester) biospheres. After a single dose administered subcutaneously to healthy volunteers, IFN-α2b was detectable in the serum at 14 days and had few side effects.[48] In a phase IIa open-labeled, dose-ranging trial, 32 patients were randomized to receive subcutaneous injections of Locteron every 14 days for 12 weeks in dose cohorts of 160, 320, 480, and 640 mcg along with weight-based doses of ribavirin.[49] A dose-dependent antiviral effect was present, with all patients in the highest dosing cohorts (n =16) achieving an early viral response.

Another drug in development is IFN-α2bXL, which uses the Medusa polymer technology to provide sustained release of the drug. Medusa (Flamel Technologies) is a self-assembled poly-amino acid nanoparticle system that allows noncovalent capture and subsequent delivery of peptide or protein drugs. The objective of IFN-α2bXL is to decrease the toxicities associated with peak levels of IFN while improving efficacy. A phase Ib randomized, controlled study dosed IFN-α2bXL once a week for 2 doses at 18 and 27 MIU and compared the antiviral effects to PEG-IFN-α2b 1.5 μg/kg/wk. IFN-α2bXL exhibited dose-dependent anti-HCV activity, with the 27 MIU dose comparing favorably with PEG-IFN-α2b.[50] There were fewer adverse events reported in the IFN-α2bXL group, providing further rationale for moving forward to phase II trials.

OTHER AGENTS TO STIMULATE INDUCTION OF IFN-α

Plasmacytoid dendritic cells (PDCs) are highly specialized immune cells capable of producing large amounts of type I and type III interferon in response to a viral infection. The response is mediated through toll-like receptor (TLR) signaling pathways, TLR7 and TLR9, which recognize the RNA and DNA of the invading pathogen.[51] In theory, stimulating PDCs directly may allow a localized, endogenous IFN release at the site of infection and also enhance the immune response to HCV. Compounds that take advantage of this pathway to stimulate the innate and adaptive immune response have been evaluated in early HCV trials, however, the results have thus far been disappointing.[52,53]

OTHER TYPES OF IFN

All of the previously mentioned therapeutic IFNs in development are a variation of IFN-α in an effort to improve on side effects, delivery, and efficacy. However, IFN-α is part of a much larger family of innate cytokines called type I IFNs, which are defined by the type of cell surface receptor with which they interact.[54] Type I IFNs also include IFN-β (beta), IFN-ω (omega), IFN-γ (gamma), and a more recently described IFN-λ (lambda).

IFN-β

Although IFN-α and IFN-β bind to the same receptor, in vitro data suggest the downstream signal responses generated by IFN-β are different from IFN-α, and distinct patterns of gene expression are seen.[55,56] The clinical efficacy of IFN-β1a has been explored in several patient populations across a range of dosing strengths, methods of administration (intravenous, subcutaneous, and intramuscular) and duration of treatment.[57–62] An interesting finding from an international, multicenter phase II study in IFN-α nonresponders was that Chinese patients were more likely to achieve an SVR than other races (OR 12.3; 95% CI 2.6–59.3).[63] Subsequent results from a Chinese HCV-naive population treated either with IFN-β1a monotherapy or IFN-β1a in combination with ribavirin are encouraging. After 24 weeks, an SVR was achieved in more patients treated with combination therapy than in those treated with monotherapy (58% versus 27%, $P < .001$).[64] The reported SVR with 24 weeks of combination therapy is comparable with the studies using 48 weeks of PEG-IFN-α and ribavirin.[12–14] This shorter duration of therapy could be a major advantage over the current standard of care, although randomized controlled trials comparing efficacy with PEG-IFN/RBV are lacking. Unfortunately, the drug must be administered 3 times per week in its current formulation. More extensive evaluation of its clinical efficacy in a broader population and under controlled trials is necessary before IFN-β1a is likely to be used in routine clinical practice outside of Asia.

IFN-ω

IFN-ω shares a similar amino acid sequence and binds to the same receptor as IFN-α activating similar antiviral pathways. In the HCV replicon system, a fully glycosylated IFN-ω derived from Chinese hamster ovary (CHO) cells showed more potent antiviral activity than either IFN-α or the nonglycosylated IFN-ω, suggesting that glycosylation has an important effect on activity.[65] In addition, IFN-ω induced similar transcription factors as IFN-α. A dose-ranging (15–120 mcg administered subcutaneously 3 times per week for 12 weeks) phase II study in 90 HCV treatment-naive patients demonstrated dose-related anti-HCV activity across genotypes 1 to 4 and a typical adverse event profile related to IFN.[66] Results from a phase II study of 102 HCV genotype 1 treatment-naive patients treated with IFN-ω 25 mcg daily for 48 weeks either alone or in combination with ribavirin 1000-1200 mg have been reported.[67,68] An early viral response (EVR) was seen in 60% of those treated with IFN-ω alone and 83.6% of those treated with IFN-ω and ribavirin. The SVR for combination therapy was 36% versus 6% with monotherapy.[67] Only 2 patients discontinued drug secondary to adverse events. The obvious disadvantage for the current formulation of IFN-ω is the requirement for daily dosing. To overcome this problem, IFN-ω is now being studied using a proprietary delivery system (DUROS device) that can be implanted subcutaneously. The proposed advantage is constant delivery of therapeutic levels of IFN-ω, which could improve the side effect profile associated with peaks/troughs of IFN and improve efficacy from limited trough levels and associated viral breakthrough. The current delivery system being investigated would supply 3 months of IFN with a single implantation.

IFN-γ

The only known type II IFN is IFN-γ. The function of IFN-γ is considered to be as an immune modulator and mediator of T cell activity. The production of IFN-γ is limited to cells of the immune system, such as T cells, natural killer cells (NK), and macrophages, after activation by a foreign antigen in the early stages of the innate immune response.[69] In vitro studies with IFN-γ demonstrate amplified NK cell activation and induction of a Th1 response when paired with IFN-α, both of which are believed to be involved in HCV clearance.[70] In addition to its immunomodulatory properties, IFN-γ can directly inhibit HCV replication in a cell culture model.[71,72] For these reasons, it was felt to be an attractive alternative to IFN-α for the treatment of chronic

HCV. A pilot study was conducted in a group of nonresponders to previous IFN-α treatment. A range of doses (100–400 μg) were administered 3 times per week for 4 weeks, and although it was well tolerated, no decrease in HCV RNA levels was demonstrated.[73] IFN-γ was also studied as a potential antifibrotic/maintenance therapy. A large, phase IIb multicenter, randomized, controlled trial using hepatic fibrosis as the primary end point in patients with advanced fibrosis or cirrhosis due to HCV has been completed and did not show any benefit of IFN-γ in reaching this end point.[74] Despite delivering prolonged, high doses of IFN-γ, no significant antiviral activity was observed. These results illustrate that significant in vitro activity does not always translate to clinical applicability, and IFN- γ is unlikely to find a role in HCV treatment regimens.

IFN-λ

IFN-λ (IFN-λ1, also known as IL-29) is part of a recently described family of IFN-related cytokines.[75] It induces the expression of genes normally activated by IFN-α by binding to a unique receptor that is primarily expressed on epithelial-derived cells, including hepatocytes.[76] IFN-λ1 also has antiviral activity similar to IFN-α, and has been shown to inhibit HCV replication in vitro.[76,77] A pegylated version of IFN-λ1 (PEG-rIL-29) is in early development. The potential therapeutic advantage of using this pathway relates to the limited expression of the IFN-λ1 receptor on hematopoetic and neuronal cells, which should minimize the expected side effects of IFN-α while maintaining anti-HCV activity. Phase Ia data suggest that PEG-rIL-29 is safe and well tolerated up to doses of 5 μg/kg without flu-like symptoms or changes in hematologic parameters.[78] A phase Ib dose and schedule escalation trial is underway in HCV genotype 1 relapsers. Interim data using PEG-rIL-29 as a single agent showed antiviral activity is best at weekly doses of 1.5 μg/kg. Neutropenia, thrombocytopenia, or anemia were not reported and minimal constitutional symptoms were present.[79] The final data from this early study will include 2 cohorts using combination therapy with ribavirin. Cell culture data also suggest that IL-29 and IFN-α have an additive antiviral effect on HCV replication and that IL-29 and IFN-γ have a synergistic effect,[80] suggesting a potential role for combination therapy to achieve additional antiviral activity. In summary, the early robust antiviral activity of IFN-λ1, along with its potential for a favorable side effect profile will make this an attractive IFN to explore in combination with STAT-C agents.

SUMMARY

Despite over 2 decades of use for HCV treatment, there continues to be great interest in drug development for new types of IFN-α that offer therapeutic advantages over the current standard of care. IFN-α will continue to be the backbone of HCV treatment for the foreseeable future, although targeted small molecule therapy with potent antiviral activity will change the landscape of treatment in the next few years. How these newly developed IFNs will fit into treatment regimens remains to be seen. Any IFN that offers improved efficacy with limited side effects would be a welcome addition to the current therapeutic armamentarium for HCV.

REFERENCES

1. Isaacs A, Lindenmann J. Virus interference. I. The interferon. Proc R Soc Lond B Biol Sci 1957;147:258–67.
2. Hoofnagle JH, Mullen KD, Jones DB, et al. Treatment of chronic non-A, non-B hepatitis with recombinant human alpha interferon. A preliminary report. N Engl J Med 1986;315:1575–8.

3. Pawlotsky J-M. Therapy of hepatitis C: From empiricism to eradication. Hepatology 2006;43:S207–20.
4. Di Bisceglie AM, Hoofnagle JH. Optimal therapy of hepatitis C. Hepatology 2002; 36:S121–7.
5. National Institutes of Health Consensus Development Conference Panel statement: management of hepatitis C. Hepatology 1997;26:2S–10S.
6. McHutchison JG, Gordon SC, Schiff ER, et al. Interferon alfa-2b alone or in combination with ribavirin as initial treatment for chronic hepatitis C. Hepatitis Interventional Therapy Group. N Engl J Med 1998;339:1485–92.
7. Poynard T, Marcellin P, Lee SS, et al. Randomised trial of interferon alpha2b plus ribavirin for 48 weeks or for 24 weeks versus interferon alpha2b plus placebo for 48 weeks for treatment of chronic infection with hepatitis C virus. International Hepatitis Interventional Therapy Group (IHIT). Lancet 1998;352:1426–32.
8. Reddy KR. Development and pharmacokinetics and pharmacodynamics of pegylated interferon alfa-2a (40 kD). Semin Liver Dis 2004;24(Suppl 2):33–8.
9. Zeuzem S, Teuber G, Naumann U, et al. Randomized, double-blind, placebo-controlled trial of interferon alfa2a with and without amantadine as initial treatment for chronic hepatitis C. Hepatology 2000;32:835–41.
10. Heathcote EJ, Shiffman ML, Cooksley WG, et al. Peginterferon alfa-2a in patients with chronic hepatitis C and cirrhosis. N Engl J Med 2000;343:1673–80.
11. Lindsay KL, Trepo C, Heintges T, et al. A randomized, double-blind trial comparing pegylated interferon alfa-2b to interferon alfa-2b as initial treatment for chronic hepatitis C. Hepatology 2001;34:395–403.
12. Fried MW, Shiffman ML, Reddy KR, et al. Peginterferon alfa-2a plus ribavirin for chronic hepatitis C virus infection. N Engl J Med 2002;347:975–82.
13. Manns MP, McHutchison JG, Gordon SC, et al. Peginterferon alfa-2b plus ribavirin compared with interferon alfa-2b plus ribavirin for initial treatment of chronic hepatitis C: a randomised trial. Lancet 2001;358:958–65.
14. Hadziyannis SJ. Peginterferon-alpha2a and ribavirin combination therapy in chronic hepatitis C: a randomized study of treatment duration and ribavirin dose. Ann Intern Med 2004;140:346–55.
15. Russo MW, Fried MW. Side effects of therapy for chronic hepatitis C. Gastroenterology 2003;124:1711–9.
16. Keeffe EB, Kowdley KV. Hematologic side effects of PEG interferon and ribavirin. Management with growth factors. J Clin Gastroenterol 2005;39:S1–2.
17. Hassanein T, Cooksley G, Sulkowski M, et al. The impact of peginterferon alfa-2a plus ribavirin combination therapy on health-related quality of life in chronic hepatitis C. J Hepatol 2004;40:675–81.
18. Davis GL. New therapies: oral inhibitors and immune modulators. Clin Liver Dis 2006;10:867–80.
19. Pawlotsky J-M, Chevaliez S, McHutchison JG. The hepatitis C virus life cycle as a target for new antiviral therapies. Gastroenterology 2007;132:1979–98.
20. De Francesco R, Migliaccio G. Challenges and successes in developing new therapies for hepatitis C. Nature 2005;436:953–60.
21. Zeuzem S, Nelson DR, Marcellin P. Dynamic evolution of therapy for chronic hepatitis C: how will novel agents be incorporated into the standard of care? Antivir Ther 2008;13:747–60.
22. McHutchison JG, Everson GT, Gordon SC, et al. Telaprevir with peginterferon and ribavirin for chronic HCV genotype 1 infection. N Engl J Med 2009;360:1827–38.
23. Feld JJ, Hoofnagle JH. Mechanism of action of interferon and ribavirin in treatment of hepatitis C. Nature 2005;436:967–72.

24. Subramanian GM, Fiscella M, Lamouse-Smith A, et al. Albinterferon [alpha]-2b: a genetic fusion protein for the treatment of chronic hepatitis C. Nat Biotechnol 2007;25:1411–9.
25. Liu C, Zhu H, Subramanian GM, et al. Anti-hepatitis C virus activity of albinterferon alfa-2b in cell culture. Hepatol Res 2007;37:941–7.
26. Osborn BL, Olsen HS, Nardelli B, et al. Pharmacokinetic and pharmacodynamic studies of a human serum albumin-interferon-alpha fusion protein in cynomolgus monkeys. J Pharmacol Exp Ther 2002;303:540–8.
27. Balan V, Nelson DR, Sulkowski MS, et al. A Phase I/II study evaluating escalating doses of recombinant human albumin-interferon-alpha fusion protein in chronic hepatitis C patients who have failed previous interferon-alpha-based therapy. Antivir Ther 2006;11:35–45.
28. Balan V, Nelson DR, Sulkowski MS, et al. Modulation of interferon-specific gene expression by albumin-interferon-alpha in interferon-alpha-experienced patients with chronic hepatitis C. Antivir Ther 2006;11:901–8.
29. Bain VG, Kaita KD, Yoshida EM, et al. A phase 2 study to evaluate the antiviral activity, safety, and pharmacokinetics of recombinant human albumin-interferon alfa fusion protein in genotype 1 chronic hepatitis C patients. J Hepatol 2006; 44:671–8.
30. Zeuzem S, Yoshida EM, Benhamou Y, et al. Albinterferon alfa-2b dosed every two or four weeks in interferon-naïve patients with genotype 1 chronic hepatitis C. Hepatology 2008;48:407–17.
31. Nelson DR, Rustgi V, Balan V, et al. Safety and antiviral activity of albinterferon alfa-2b in prior interferon nonresponders with chronic hepatitis C. Clin Gastroenterol Hepatol 2009;7:212–8.
32. Zeuzem S, Sulkowski M, Lawitz E, et al. Efficacy and safety of albinterferon alfa-2b in combination with ribavirin in treatment-naïve patients with chronic hepatitis C genotype 1 [oral presentation]. 44th Annual Meeting of the European Association for the Study of the Liver. April 25, 2009.
33. Nelson D, Benhamou Y, Chuang WL, et al. Efficacy and safety results of albinterferon alfa-2b in combination with ribavirin in treatment-naïve patients with chronic hepatitis C genotype 2 or 3 [oral presentation]. 44th Annual Meeting of the European Association for the Study of the Liver. April 25, 2009.
34. Keeffe EB, Hollinger FB, Group CIS. Therapy of hepatitis C: consensus interferon trials. Hepatology 1997;26:101S–7S.
35. Blatt LM, Davis JM, Klein SB, et al. The biologic activity and molecular characterization of a novel synthetic interferon-alpha species, consensus interferon. J Interferon Cytokine Res 1996;16:489–99.
36. Ozes ON, Reiter Z, Klein S, et al. A comparison of interferon-Con1 with natural recombinant interferons-alpha: antiviral, antiproliferative, and natural killer-inducing activities. J Interferon Res 1992;12:55–9.
37. Tong MJ, Reddy KR, Lee WM, et al. Treatment of chronic hepatitis C with consensus interferon: a multicenter, randomized, controlled trial. Consensus Interferon Study Group. Hepatology 1997;26:747–54.
38. Sjogren MH, Sjogren R Jr, Lyons MF, et al. Antiviral response of HCV genotype 1 to consensus interferon and ribavirin versus pegylated interferon and ribavirin. Dig Dis Sci 2007;52:1540–7.
39. Blatt LM, Cheung E, Radhakrishma R, et al. A phase 1, single-blind, dose-escalating study of the safety and pharmacokinetics of a single injection of pegylated interferon alfacon-1 in healthy volunteers [abstract]. Gastroenterology 2005;128: S713.

40. Leevy CB. Consensus interferon and ribavirin in patients with chronic hepatitis C who were nonresponders to pegylated interferon alfa-2b and ribavirin. Dig Dis Sci 2008;53:1961–6.
41. Miglioresi L, Bacosi M, Russo F, et al. Consensus interferon versus interferon-alpha 2b plus ribavirin in patients with relapsing HCV infection. Hepatol Res 2003;27:253–9.
42. Graddis TJ, Remmele RL Jr, McGrew JT. Designing proteins that work using recombinant technologies. Curr Pharm Biotechnol 2002;3:285–97.
43. Brideau-Andersen AD, Huang X, Sun S-CC, et al. Directed evolution of gene-shuffled IFN-α molecules with activity profiles tailored for treatment of chronic viral diseases. Proc Natl Acad Sci U S A 2007;104:8269–74.
44. Shriver Z, Raguram S, Sasisekharan R. Glycomics: a pathway to a class of new and improved therapeutics. Nat Rev Drug Discov 2004;3:863–73.
45. Bailon P, Palleroni A, Schaffer CA, et al. Rational design of a potent, long-lasting form of interferon: a 40 kDa branched polyethylene glycol-conjugated interferon alpha-2a for the treatment of hepatitis C. Bioconjug Chem 2001;12:195–202.
46. Foser S, Schacher A, Weyer KA, et al. Isolation, structural characterization, and antiviral activity of positional isomers of monopegylated interferon alpha-2a (PEGASYS). Protein Expr Purif 2003;30:78–87.
47. Blatt LM, Seiwert S, Beigleman L. Development of novel hyperglycosylated type 1 interferons: a strategy to improve PK performance without loss of biological potency [abstract]. J Hepatol 2008;48:S10.
48. De Leede LG, Humphries JE, Bechet AC, et al. Novel controlled-release Lemna-derived IFN-alpha2b (Locteron): pharmacokinetics, pharmacodynamics, and tolerability in a phase I clinical trial. J Interferon Cytokine Res 2008;28:113–22.
49. Herrmann E, Zeuzem S, Dzyublyk I, et al. Viral kinetics during treatment with a controlled-release recombinant interferon alfa 2b in genotype 1 chronic hepatitis C patients [abstract]. J Hepatol 2008;48:S318.
50. Trepo C, Guest M, Meyrueix R, et al. Evaluation of antiviral activity and tolerance of a novel sustained release interferon-alpha-2b (IFN-Alpha-2bXL) compared to pegylated interferon-alpha-2b (PEG-IFN-alpha-2b): a phase 1b trial in HCV patients [abstract]. J Hepatol 2008;48:S28.
51. Guiducci C, Coffman RL, Barrat FJ. Signalling pathways leading to IFN-alpha production in human plasmacytoid dendritic cell and the possible use of agonists or antagonists of TLR7 and TLR9 in clinical indications. J Intern Med 2009;265:43–57.
52. Vicari AP, Schmalbach T, Lekstrom-Himes J, et al. Safety, pharmacokinetics, and immune effects in normal volunteers of CPG 10101(ACTILON), an investigational synthetic TLR agonist. Antivir Ther 2007;12:741–51.
53. McHutchison JG, Bacon BR, Gordon SC, et al. Phase 1B, randomized, double-blind, dose-escalation trial of CPG 10101 in patients with chronic hepatitis C virus. Hepatology 2007;46:1341–9.
54. Chevaliez S, Pawlotsky J-M. Interferon-based therapy of hepatitis C. Adv Drug Deliv Rev 2007;59:1222–41.
55. Platanias LC, Uddin S, Colamonici OR. Tyrosine phosphorylation of the alpha and beta subunits of the type I interferon receptor. Interferon-beta selectively induces tyrosine phosphorylation of an alpha subunit-associated protein. J Biol Chem 1994;269:17761–4.
56. Der SD, Zhou A, Williams BR, et al. Identification of genes differentially regulated by interferon alpha, beta, or gamma using oligonucleotide arrays. Proc Natl Acad Sci U S A 1998;95:15623–8.

57. Habersetzer F, Boyer N, Marcellin P, et al. A pilot study of recombinant interferon beta-1a for the treatment of chronic hepatitis C. Liver 2000;20:437–41.
58. Pellicano R, Craxi A, Almasio PL, et al. Interferon beta-1a alone or in combination with ribavirin: a randomized trial to compare efficacy and safety in chronic hepatitis C. World J Gastroenterol 2005;11:4484–9.
59. Han Q, Liu Z, Kang W, et al. Interferon beta 1a versus interferon beta 1a plus ribavirin for the treatment of chronic hepatitis C in Chinese patients: a randomized, placebo-controlled trial. Dig Dis Sci 2008;53:2238–45.
60. Kobayashi Y, Watanabe S, Konishi M, et al. Quantitation and typing of serum hepatitis C virus RNA in patients with chronic hepatitis C treated with interferon-beta. Hepatology 1993;18:1319–25.
61. Pellicano R, Palmas F, Cariti G, et al. Re-treatment with interferon-beta of patients with chronic hepatitis C virus infection. Eur J Gastroenterol Hepatol 2002;14: 1377–82.
62. Festi D, Sandri L, Mazzella G, et al. Safety of interferon beta treatment for chronic HCV hepatitis. World J Gastroenterol 2004;10:12–6.
63. Cheng PN, Marcellin P, Bacon B, et al. Racial differences in responses to interferon-beta-1a in chronic hepatitis C unresponsive to interferon-alpha: a better response in Chinese patients. J Viral Hepat 2004;11:418–26.
64. Chan HL, Ren H, Chow WC, et al. Group Ib-aHCS. Randomized trial of interferon beta-1a with or without ribavirin in Asian patients with chronic hepatitis C. Hepatology 2007;46:315–23.
65. Buckwold VE, Wei J, Huang Z, et al. Antiviral activity of CHO-SS cell-derived human omega interferon and other human interferons against HCV RNA replicons and related viruses. Antiviral Res 2007;73:118–25.
66. Plauth M, Meisel H, Langecker P, et al. Open-label study of omega interferon in previously untreated HCV-infected patients [abstract]. J Hepatol 2002;36:S125.
67. Novozhenov V, Zakharova N, Vinogradova E, et al. Phase 2 study of omega interferon alone or in combination with ribavirin in subjects with chronic hepatitis C genotype-1 infection [abstract]. J Hepatol 2007;46:S8.
68. Gorbakov V, Kim H, Oronsky B, et al. HCV RNA results from a phase II, randomized, open-label study of omega interferon with or without ribavirin in IFN-naive genotype 1 chronic HCV patients [abstract]. Hepatology 2005;42:S705.
69. Boehm U, Klamp T, Groot M, et al. Cellular responses to interferon-gamma. Annu Rev Immunol 1997;15:749–95.
70. Wang T, Blatt LM, Seiwert SD. Immunomodulatory activities of IFN-gamma1b in combination with type I IFN: implications for the use of IFN-gamma1b in the treatment of chronic HCV infections. J Interferon Cytokine Res 2006;26:473–83.
71. Dash S, Prabhu R, Hazari S, et al. Interferons alpha, beta, gamma each inhibit hepatitis C virus replication at the level of internal ribosome entry site-mediated translation. Liver Int 2005;25:580–94.
72. Frese M, Schwarzle V, Barth K, et al. Interferon-gamma inhibits replication of subgenomic and genomic hepatitis C virus RNAs. Hepatology 2002;35:694–703.
73. Soza A, Heller T, Ghany M, et al. Pilot study of interferon gamma for chronic hepatitis C. J Hepatol 2005;43:67–71.
74. Pockros PJ, Jeffers L, Afdhal N, et al. Final results of a double-blind, placebo-controlled trial of the antifibrotic efficacy of interferon-gamma1b in chronic hepatitis C patients with advanced fibrosis or cirrhosis. Hepatology 2007;45:569–78.
75. Sheppard P, Kindsvogel W, Xu W, et al. IL-28, IL-29 and their class II cytokine receptor IL-28R. Nat Immunol 2003;4:63–8.

76. Doyle SE, Schreckhise H, Khuu-Duong K, et al. Interleukin-29 uses a type 1 interferon-like program to promote antiviral responses in human hepatocytes. Hepatology 2006;44:896–906.
77. Marcello T, Grakoui A, Barba-Spaeth G, et al. Interferons alpha and lambda inhibit hepatitis C virus replication with distinct signal transduction and gene regulation kinetics. Gastroenterology 2006;131:1887–98.
78. Hausman D, Freeman J, Souza S, et al. A phase 1, randomized, blinded, placebo controlled, single-dose, dose escalation study of PEG-interferon lambda (PEG-rIL-29) in healthy subjects. HEP DART Annual Meeting, Maui, Hawaii, December 9–13, 2007.
79. Lawitz E, Zaman A, Muir A, et al. Interim results from a phase 1b dose escalation study of 4 weeks of PEG-interferon lambda(PEG-rIL-29) treatment in subjects with hepatitis C virus genotype 1 with prior virologic response and relapse to PEG-interferon alfa and ribavirin [abstract]. Hepatology 2008;48:S385.
80. Pagliaccetti N, Eduardo R, Kleinstein S, et al. Interleukin-29 functions cooperatively with interferon to induce antiviral gene expression and inhibit hepatitis C virus replication. J Biol Chem 2008;283:30079–89.

Antifibrotics for Chronic Hepatitis C

Paul J. Pockros, MD*

KEYWORDS

• Hepatitis C virus • Interferon-gamma 1b • Antifibrotics
• Caspase inhibitors • Long-term pegylated interferons

Fibrosis is currently viewed as a dynamic rather than a static process; extracellular matrix is constantly being laid down and resorbed, and the progressive accumulation of fibrous tissue is believed to represent a relative imbalance between profibrotic and antifibrotic processes.[1] The central cells involved in the pathogenesis of hepatic fibrosis are hepatic stellate cells (HSCs), also known as lipocytes, fat-storing cells, Ito cells, or myofibroblasts.[2] Cytokines play major roles at all stages in the development of fibrosis, including hepatocyte injury, inflammatory response, altered function of sinusoidal cells (particularly HSCs), extracellular matrix accumulation, and matrix degradation. Cytokines play an especially important role in perpetuating and modulating the effects of activated HSCs. In experimental models of fibrosis, transforming growth factor-β (TGF-β) has been shown to play a key role in stimulating and maintaining the fibrogenic process. In the liver, TGF-β stimulates the expression of extracellular matrix proteins and collagen, inhibits collagenases, and promotes the activation of fat-storing HSCs toward a myofibroblast phenotype.[3] In addition, inhibition of TGF-β is effective in preventing fibrosis and preserving organ function.[1]

Antifibrotic agents developed or tested for treatment of chronic hepatitis C generally are targeted toward HSCs, TGF-β, the inflammatory response, or extracellular matrix accumulation. Although several agents have been or are being currently studied in this indication, to date none have proved to be effective. There is a clear need for drugs which inhibit or reverse hepatic fibrosis, as these would be immediately applicable to patients who have failed antiviral therapy or have contraindications to antiviral therapy such as those with decompensated liver disease or renal failure. These drugs would be important adjuncts in patients in whom rapid development of fibrosis threatens liver function before antiviral therapies may be effective, such as those who are coinfected with hepatitis C virus (HCV) and HIV or those who have cholestatic fibrosing hepatitis due to recurrent HCV post-transplantation. A major impediment in the development of new drugs in this field has been the inability to identify reasonable

* Division of Gastroenterology and Hepatology, The Scripps Research Institute, 10666 North Torrey Pines Road, La Jolla, CA 92037, USA.
E-mail address: pockros.paul@scrippshealth.org

Clin Liver Dis 13 (2009) 365–373
doi:10.1016/j.cld.2009.05.005
liver.theclinics.com
1089-3261/09/$ – see front matter

histologic or clinical end points within a reasonable period of study. This factor has contributed to the failure of several the compounds discussed herein. **Box 1** lists several key agents studied or being studied as antifibrotics for HCV. There are only limited published data available for most of these compounds so only those best studied to date are discussed in this article.

INTERFERON-GAMMA

Interferon-gamma (IFN-γ) has been shown to profoundly affect the fibrotic process. IFN-γ has been found to be a key counterregulatory antifibrotic cytokine balancing

Box 1
Experimental antifibrotic agents

5-Lipoxygenase-activating protein inhibitors
Interferon-γ, -α
AA861 mycophenolate
Angiotensin-converting enzyme inhibitors
Octreotide
Anti-a1 integrin
Pentoxifylline
Arginine-glycine-aspartate peptides
Caspase inhibitors
Peroxisome proliferator-activated receptor ligands
Estradiol
Prostaglandins, prostaglandin E2
Endothelin A receptor antagonists
Quercetin
Farnesoid X receptor agonists
Rapamycin
Glycyrrhizin/*Salvia miltiorrhiza*
Retinoic acid
Halofuginone Sho-saiko-to (TJ-9)
Hepatocyte growth factor
Soluble platelet-derived growth factor antagonists
High-dose antioxidants (silymarin)
Soluble type II fusion molecule
HOE 77a
Transforming growth factor β-receptor blockade
Interleukin-1 antagonists

Data from McHutchison JG, Poynard T, Afdhal N, et al. Fibrosis as an end point for clinical trials in liver disease: a consensus report of the International Fibrosis Group. Clin Gastroenterol Hepatol 2006;4(10):1215.

the activity of TGF-β.[4] IFN-γ inhibits the interaction of downstream proteins that are normally activated following the binding of TGF-β to its cellular receptor. As a result, transcriptional responses to TGF-β signaling are inhibited. The degree of inhibition is dependent in part on the relative amounts of TGF-β and IFN-γ, indicating that the extent of inhibition (or activation) of TGF-β responsive genes may be determined by the balance of TGF-β and IFN-γ signals. This provides a theoretical rationale for the use of pharmacologic doses of IFN-γ even in those settings in which there are elevated levels of intrinsic IFN-γ and TGF-β.[5]

Experimental data from in vitro studies, studies in animal models of liver fibrosis, and studies in humans with idiopathic pulmonary fibrosis (IPF) all support a potential therapeutic role for IFN-γ1b in the inhibition of fibrosis in the liver and other organs.[1–7] Studies of the in vitro effects of IFN-γ on cultured murine and human HSC consistently demonstrate that IFN-γ inhibits the proliferation and culture-induced activation of these cells. These studies also demonstrate that IFN-γ inhibits the expression of mRNA encoding extracellular matrix proteins, leading to a significant reduction in the production of extracellular matrix proteins. Several studies have been published on the antifibrotic activity of IFN-γ in animal models of liver fibrosis. These studies consistently demonstrate that IFN-γ administered during the period of hepatic injury is capable of reducing the quantity of extracellular matrix and of reducing the degree of histologically evident fibrosis present in the liver.

Two studies have provided data relevant to assessing the potential antifibrotic effects of IFN-γ1b in humans. The first was a randomized controlled study on the effects of IFN in IPF, a progressive fibrosing disease of unknown cause with a mean survival time of 2 to 4 years. Based on the antifibrotic effects of IFN-γ demonstrated in in vitro and in vivo animal models, Ziesche and colleagues[6] conducted an open-label, randomized, controlled trial comparing the safety and efficacy of IFN-γ1b plus low-dose prednisolone (n = 9) with that of prednisolone alone (n = 9) in patients with IPF confirmed by biopsy or by high-resolution computed tomography (HRCT). Over the course of the study, all patients treated with IFN-γ1b showed improvement in pulmonary function. In contrast, patients treated with prednisolone alone showed deterioration in their condition. The differences between the 2 groups at 12 months were statistically significant for total lung capacity (TLC) ($P<.001$ for difference between groups) and for PaO_2 at rest and on maximal exertion (both $P<.001$ for difference in change from baseline).

The second study was a small pilot study comparing IFN-γ1b with IFN-α in patients with chronic hepatitis C in which paired biopsies were obtained in a subset of patients. Saez-Royuela and colleagues[7] conducted a randomized controlled pilot study of IFN-α2c and IFN-γ1b in 30 adults with chronic hepatitis C with persistently elevated serum alanine aminotransferase (ALT) levels. There was a trend toward a decrease in the fibrosis score in IFN-γ1b recipients with a reduction in fibrosis from 1.2 ± 1.0 to 0.7 ± 1.0 on the Knodell fibrosis score. Combined with the findings from the trial in IPF, these studies provided a rationale to study hepatic fibrosis in a larger group of patients with HCV.

A large, multicenter, randomized controlled trial (AEGIS) using hepatic fibrosis as the primary end point in patients with advanced fibrosis or cirrhosis due to HCV enrolled a total of 502 patients with compensated liver disease and an Ishak fibrosis score of 4 to 6 and 488 of these patients received subcutaneous injections of IFN-γ1b 100 μg (group 1, n = 169), IFN-γ1b 200 μg (group 2, n = 157), or placebo (group 3, n = 162) 3 times a week for 48 weeks.[8] Most patients (83.6%) had cirrhosis at baseline (Ishak score 5 or 6). Post-treatment liver biopsies were assessed in a blinded fashion for a reduction of 1 or more Ishak points (primary end point). Four hundred and twenty patients with pretreatment and post-treatment liver biopsies were evaluable and showed no improvement in Ishak score between the 3 treatment groups (12.1%, 12.4%, and 16% of patients in groups 1, 2, and 3, respectively; $P > .05$). There were similar numbers of deaths in all 3 arms (5, 5, and 4, respectively), and most were related to complications of cirrhosis. The investigators concluded that IFN-γ1b therapy was not able to reverse fibrosis in patients with advanced liver disease for 1 year, and that perhaps less advanced disease should be considered for future studies with IFN-γ1b or other antifibrotic agents.

Two smaller studies using IFN-γ for HCV also failed to show any benefit in fibrosis progression or a sustained antiviral effect, suggesting that this compound will not likely be developed any further for the indication of HCV.[9,10] IFN-γ had been studied earlier for chronic hepatitis B (HBV) and failed to show antiviral efficacy.[11,12] A subsequent trial in HBV showed a mild antiviral effect and antifibrotic benefit, although the study was not powered to make definitive conclusions.[13] Further development of IFN-γ for HBV or HCV is not currently underway.

Fibrosis progression in chronic liver disease has usually been evaluated by liver biopsy using insensitive semiquantitative numerical scores. An alternative to this is to measure fibrous tissue quantitatively using morphometric image analysis. Morphometry was used to quantify the amount of fibrous tissue in liver biopsies performed at baseline and after 48 weeks in 245 patients in the large IFN-γ1b trial who had paired unfragmented, adequate-sized specimens.[14] Because no effect of the drug on fibrosis was found in the trial, data from all 245 patients could be combined for analysis. At baseline, 78% had cirrhosis and 22% had bridging fibrosis. The mean morphometrically determined collagen content increased by 58% between baseline and 48 weeks. There were statistically significant but weak correlations of fibrosis with platelet count, albumin, bilirubin, international normalized ratio (INR), and hyaluronic acid, but changes in these did not correlate with or predict changes in fibrosis in the liver biopsy. The investigators concluded that in advanced chronic hepatitis C, fibrosis increases at a rapid pace, which can only be detected by morphometry (**Fig. 1**). A subsequent consensus report suggested that this technique be used in future therapeutic trials of agents to inhibit fibrosis progression.[15]

LONG-TERM PEGYLATED INTERFERON STUDIES ON LIVER FIBROSIS

A sensible approach to slow or reverse hepatic fibrosis in HCV would be to attempt to suppress viral replication and intrahepatic inflammation. The ideal study would use clinical end points such as death, transplantation, variceal hemorrhage, or hepatocellular carcinoma. Measurement of these end points requires large sample sizes and long follow-up periods, caveats that limit these studies to federal funding or major industry commitments. Three long-term studies of liver fibrosis in patients with advanced HCV using long-term IFN therapy have been completed and their data have been presented or published (**Table 1**). In 2008, Di Bisceglie published the long-awaited but disappointing results of the long-term Hepatitis C Antiviral Long-term Treatment against Cirrhosis (HALT-C) trial for nonresponder or relapse patients with advanced fibrosis or cirrhosis.[16] In that study, 1050 patients were followed for 3.5 years on 90 μg pegylated interferon (PegIFN)-α2a per week or no therapy after a run-in phase during which patients were treated for 20 weeks and determined to be HCV RNA positive. At the end of follow-up, equal numbers of patients had died, decompensated, or developed hepatocellular carcinoma (HCC). The increase in fibrosis measured by liver biopsy before and after treatment was identical in both

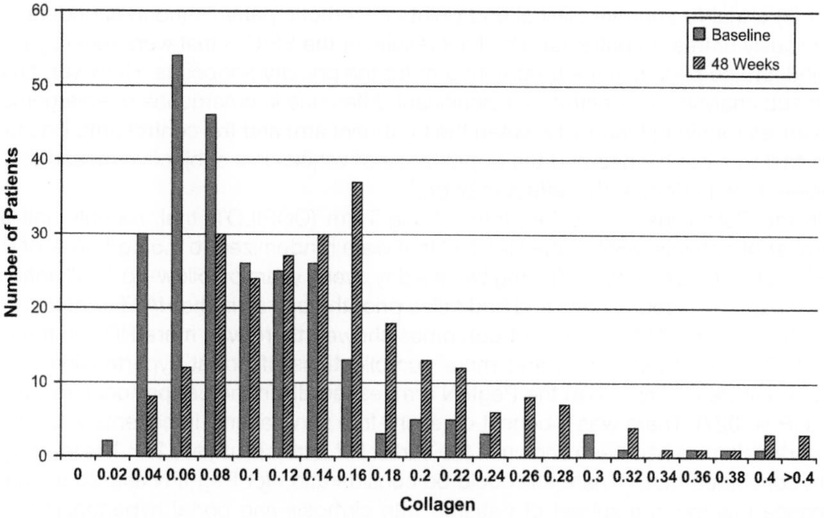

Fig. 1. Liver biopsy collagen content at baseline and after 48 weeks in 245 patients with advanced chronic hepatitis C. (*From* Goodman ZD, Becker RL, Pockros PJ, et al. Progression of fibrosis in advanced chronic hepatitis C: evaluation by morphometric image analysis. Hepatology 2007;45(4):890; with permission.)

groups. The author's conclusion was there was no proven benefit to long-term therapy with PegIFN in this population of nonresponder patients.

In the Evaluation of PegIntron in Control of hepatitis C cirrhosis (EPIC-3) study, patients with Metavir stage 2 to 4 fibrosis were randomized to receive either PegIFN-α2b at 0.5 μg/kg/wk or placebo for a 4-year period.[17] The EPIC-3 study is essentially 3 studies in 1: (1) a trial in nonresponders to previous therapy with sustained virologic response (SVR) as the clinical end point for patients with F2-4 fibrosis; (2) a trial to improve liver histology with long-term therapy in patients with F2-3 fibrosis;

Table 1
Long-term studies in liver fibrosis

	HALT-C[16]	EPIC-3[17]	COPILOT[18]
Fibrosis stage	Ishak 3–6	Metavir 2–4	Ishak 3–6
n	1000	2200 (3 studies)	600
End point	Fibrosis/clinical	Fibrosis/clinical	Clinical
Arm 1	PegIFN-α2a	PegIFN-α2b	PegIFN-α2b
—	90 μg	0.5 μg/kg	0.5 μg/kg
Arm 2	Observation	Observation	Colchicine
Run-in phase	Yes	Yes	No
Duration (years)	3.5	4	4

Abbreviations: HALT-C, Hepatitis C Antiviral Long-term Treatment against Cirrhosis trial; EPIC-3, Evaluation of PegIntron in Control of hepatitis C cirrhosis study; COPILOT, Colchicine versus PegIntron Long Term trial; IFN, interferon; Peg, pegylated.
Data from McHutchison JG, Poynard T, Afdhal N, et al. Fibrosis as an end point for clinical trials in liver disease: a consensus report of the International Fibrosis Group. Clin Gastroenterol Hepatol 2006;4(10):1219.

and (3) a trial to improve clinical end points in cirrhotic patients (nonresponders and previously untreated patients). The final results of the EPIC-3 trial were recently published and no benefit in the treatment arm for the primary endpoints. However, an ad hoc sub analysis demonstrated a significant difference in emergence or enlargement of varices requiring therapy between the treatment arm and the control arm. Because this trial was not blinded and the appearance of varices is a subjective measure, it is unclear how important this effect may be.[18]

In the Colchicine versus Peg-Intron Long Term (COPILOT) trial, roughly half the number of patients (555) of the HALT-C trial were randomized to 0.5 μg/kg/wk of PegIFN-α2b versus colchicine 0.6 mg twice a day over 4 years of follow-up.[19] All patients again had advanced fibrosis and had failed prior therapy as in the HALT-C study. The intention to treat (ITT) analysis of outcomes showed there was more HCC in the PegIFN (P = NS) treated arm and more complications of portal hypertension in the colchicine treated arm than the PegIFN arm, especially in the per protocol (PP) analysis (P = .027). There was a benefit on event-free survival only in patients with portal hypertension, as had been shown in the earlier PP analysis at year 2.[20] The investigators concluded that, "There still could be consideration for Peg-IFN alfa-2b as maintenance therapy in a subset of patients with cirrhosis and portal hypertension who failed eradication therapy. The mechanism of action we believe is mediated by the effects of portal hypertension and this seems to be more profound in the early phases of treatment."

Subsequent data from HALT-C presented by Shiffman and colleagues[21] were disappointing regarding maintenance therapy and continued HCV viral suppression. Many hoped this subgroup would benefit from long-term therapy. However, Shiffman found that a significant improvement in clinical outcomes was observed in those who achieved a profound decline in HCV RNA in the first 20 weeks of treatment (>4 log or undetectable with subsequent breakthrough or relapse) with full-dose PegIFN and ribavirin whether or not they remained on maintenance therapy. This supports the notion that viral suppression helps but only if it is attained in the first 20 weeks of treatment, again leaving slow responders or nonresponders without a benefit and showing no efficacy of long-term PegIFN. Clearly, better options are needed for these patients than maintenance therapy with PegIFN.

CASPASE INHIBITORS AS ANTIFIBROTICS

Programmed cell death or apoptosis is a tightly controlled process of cellular suicide that occurs during normal development, normal tissue turnover, and in numerous diseases.[1] In the case of inflammatory disease states such HCV, persistent inflammation may lead to disordered hepatocyte apoptosis, which in turn contributes to the progressive fibrosis.[22] Abnormally high levels of apoptotic cells are found in the liver of individuals with HCV infection and leads to stellate cell activation.[23] This in turn leads to stellate cell profibrogenic gene expression and ultimately results in increased hepatic collagen deposition.[22,23] Although inflammation may cause apoptosis, it is also known that hepatocyte apoptosis promotes inflammation, thus creating a harmful synergy of inflammation and apoptosis and eventually leading to fibrosis.[24] One treatment strategy is to reduce the inflammation and resultant fibrosis induced or mediated by hepatocyte apoptosis. Caspases, intracellular aspartate-specific cysteine proteases that function as inducers and effectors of apoptotic cell death, play a critical role in liver injury in chronic HCV infection.[25,26] Increased levels of apoptotic cells have been observed in the liver of patients with chronic HCV infection[26] and the number of apoptotic cells present in liver biopsies has been shown to correlate with the grade of inflammation.[25] Accordingly, novel agents inhibiting caspases have been tested in this clinical arena.

IDN-6556 (now known as PF-03491390) is a specific and irreversible caspase inhibitor that shows no inhibition of other classes of proteases or other enzymes or receptors.[27] IDN-6556 has been shown to have activity in animal models of liver disease in which apoptosis is believed to contribute to the pathogenesis. For instance, apoptosis has been described in a model of liver fibrosis occurring after ligation of the mouse bile duct. In this model, application of IDN-6556 suppresses apoptosis and inflammation and prevents liver fibrosis.[28] For this reason, a human study was performed to explore the effect of IDN-6556 in patients with HCV.

In a multicenter, double-blind, placebo-controlled, dose-ranging study with a 14-day dosing period, 105 patients were enrolled and 79 received active drug.[29] Eighty (80) patients had chronic hepatitis C and 25 had other liver diseases including nonalcoholic steatohepatitis (NASH), hepatitis B, primary biliary cirrhosis (PBC), and primary sclerosing cholangitis (PSC). IDN-6556 doses ranged from 5 mg to 400 mg daily given from 1 to 3 times daily. In the HCV patients all doses of IDN-6556 significantly lowered ALT and aspartate aminotransferase (AST) (P = .0041 to P<.0001 for various dosing groups in Wilcoxon tests comparing IDN-6556 with placebo) with the exception of the lowest dose (**Fig. 2**). Adverse experiences were not different between those on IDN-6556 and placebo. Mean HCV RNA levels did not show significant changes. Longer studies to assess the potential effects of IDN-6556 on liver inflammation and fibrosis were planned but drug development was halted. An area of concern for any caspase inhibitor studied in HCV is the risk of development of cancer. Because of this concern, patients were excluded from enrollment in this study if they had cirrhosis or elevation of a-fetoprotein levels, and the duration of treatment was limited to a 14 days. However, this risk clearly may cause drug developers to pause before investing large sums of money into caspase inhibitors for this indication. To our knowledge only 1 other compound (Gilead Sciences, Inc, GS-9450) is currently in development for chronic hepatitis C.[30]

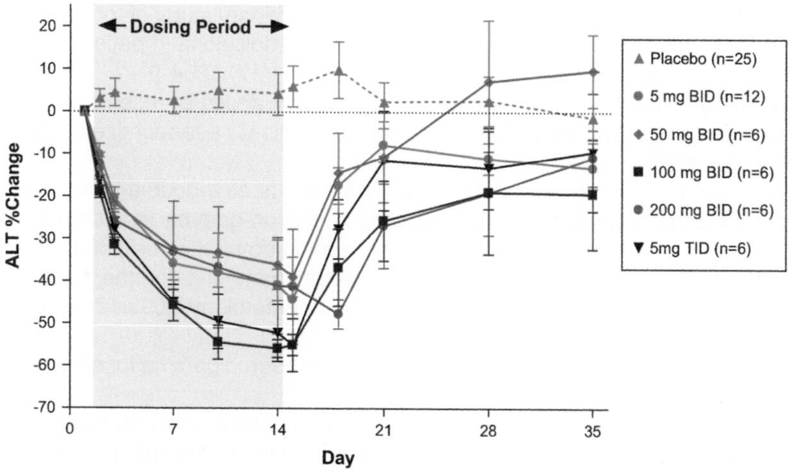

Fig. 2. ALT % change from baseline with IDN-6556, at doses twice and three times per day (means ± SEM shown). (*From* Pockros PJ, Schiff ER, Shiffman ML, et al. Oral IDN-6556, an antiapoptotic caspase inhibitor, lowers aminotransferases in patients with chronic hepatitis C. Hepatology 2007;46(2):326; with permission.)

SUMMARY

Development and testing of antifibrotic agents for the treatment of chronic hepatitis C have generally been targeted toward HSCs, TGF-β, the inflammatory response, or extracellular matrix accumulation. Although several agents such as IFN-γ, long-term PegIFN and caspase inhibitors have been studied in this indication, none have been proved to be effective to date. There is a clear need for drugs that inhibit or reverse hepatic fibrosis as these would be immediately applicable to patients who have failed antiviral therapy or have contraindications to antiviral therapy such as those with decompensated liver disease or renal failure. These drugs would be important adjuncts for patients in whom rapid development of fibrosis threatens liver function before antiviral therapies may be effective, such as those who are coinfected with HCV and HIV or those who have cholestatic fibrosing hepatitis due to recurrent HCV post-transplantation. A major impediment in the development of new drugs in this field has been the inability to identify histologic or clinical end points within a reasonable period of study. Progress will need to be made in providing suitable end points to therapy, which should then promote the development of newer agents.

REFERENCES

1. Friedman SL. Evaluation of fibrosis and hepatitis C. Am J Med 1999;107(6B): 27S–30S.
2. Nakamura T, Sakata R, Ueno T, et al. Inhibition of transforming growth factor beta prevents progression of liver fibrosis and enhances hepatocyte regeneration in dimethylnitrosamine-treated rats. Hepatology 2000;32(2):247–55.
3. Border WA, Noble NA. Transforming growth factor beta in tissue fibrosis. N Engl J Med 1994;331(19):1286–92.
4. Ulloa L, Doody J, Massague J. Inhibition of transforming growth factor-beta/SMAD signalling by the interferon-gamma/STAT pathway. Nature 1999; 397(6721):710–3.
5. Friedman SL. Molecular regulation of hepatic fibrosis, an integrated cellular response to tissue injury. J Biol Chem 2000;275:2247–50.
6. Ziesche R, Hofbauer E, Wittmann K, et al. A preliminary study of long-term treatment with interferon gamma-1b and low-dose prednisolone in patients with idiopathic pulmonary fibrosis. N Engl J Med 1999;341(17):1264–9.
7. Saez-Royuela F, Porres JC, Moreno A, et al. High doses of recombinant alpha-interferon or gamma-interferon for chronic hepatitis C: a randomized, controlled trial. Hepatology 1991;13(2):327–31.
8. Pockros PJ, Jeffers L, Afdhal N, et al. Final results of a double-blind, placebo-controlled trial of the anti-fibrotic efficacy of interferon-gamma 1b in chronic hepatitis C with advanced fibrosis or cirrhosis. Hepatology 2007;45(3):569–78.
9. Muir AJ, Sylvestre PB, Rockey DC. Interferon gamma-1 for the treatment of chronic hepatitis C infection [abstract]. Gastroenterology 2003;124(Suppl 1):A 718.
10. Soza A, Heller T, Ghany M, et al. Pilot study of interferon gamma for chronic hepatitis C. J Hepatol 2005;43(1):67–71.
11. Di Bisceglie AM, Rustgi AK, Kassianides C, et al. Therapy of chronic hepatitis B with recombinant human alpha and gamma interferon. Hepatology 1990;11(2): 266–70.
12. Kakumu S, Ishikawa T, Mizokami M, et al. Treatment with human gamma interferon of chronic hepatitis B: comparative study with alpha interferon. J Med Virol 1991;35(1):32–7.

13. Weng HL, Wang BE, Jia JD, et al. Effect of interferon gamma on hepatic fibrosis in chronic hepatitis B virus infection: a randomized controlled study. Clin Gastroenterol Hepatol 2005;3(8):819–28.
14. Goodman ZD, Becker RL, Pockros PJ, et al. Progression of fibrosis in advanced chronic hepatitis C: evaluation by morphometric image analysis. Hepatology 2007;45(4):886–94.
15. McHutchison JG, Poynard T, Afdhal N, et al. Fibrosis as an end point for clinical trials in liver disease: a consensus report of the International Fibrosis Group. Clin Gastroenterol Hepatol 2006;4(10):1214–20.
16. Di Bisceglie AM, Shiffman ML, Everson GT, et al. Prolonged therapy of advanced chronic hepatitis C with low-dose peginterferon. N Engl J Med 2008;359(23):2429–41.
17. Poynard T, Schiff E, Terg R, et al. High early viral response (EVR) with PEG-Intron/Rebetol (PR) weight based dosing (WBD) in previous interferon/ribavirin HCV treatment failures; early results of the EPIC3 trial [abstract]. Hepatology 2004; 40(Suppl 1):238A.
18. Poynard T, Colombo M, Bruix J, et al. Peginterferon alfa-2b and ribavirin: effective in patients with hepatitis C who failed interferon alfa/ribavirin therapy. Gastroenterology 2009;136(5):1618–28.
19. Afdhal NH, Levine R, Brown R Jr, et al. Colchicine versus peg-interferon alfa 2B long term therapy: results of the 4 year copilot trial [abstract]. J Hepatol 2008; 48(Suppl 2):S4.
20. Afdhal N, Frelich B, Levine R, et al. Colchicine versus PEG-Intron long term (COPILOT) trial: interim analysis of clinical outcomes at year 2 [abstract]. Hepatology 2004;40:239A.
21. Shiffman ML, Morishima C, Lindsay KL, et al. Suppression of serum HCV RNA levels during maintenance peginterferon (PEG-IFN) alfa-2a therapy and clinical outcomes in the HALT-C trial [abstract]. J Hepatol 2008;48(Suppl 2):S62.
22. Guicciardi ME, Gores GJ. Apoptosis: a mechanism of acute and chronic liver injury. Gut 2005;54(7):1024–33.
23. Bataller R, Brenner DA. Liver fibrosis. J Clin Invest 2005;115(2):209–18.
24. Canbay A, Friedman S, Gores GJ. Apoptosis: the nexus of liver injury and fibrosis. Hepatology 2004;39(2):273–8.
25. Bantel H, Lugering A, Poremba C, et al. Caspase activation correlates with the degree of inflammatory liver injury in chronic hepatitis C virus infection. Hepatology 2001;34(4 Pt 1):758–67.
26. Pianko S, Patella S, Ostapowicz G, et al. Fas-mediated hepatocyte apoptosis is increased by hepatitis C virus infection and alcohol consumption, and may be associated with hepatic fibrosis: mechanisms of liver cell injury in chronic hepatitis C virus infection. J Viral Hepat 2001;8(6):406–13.
27. Hoglen NC, Chen LS, Fisher CD, et al. Characterization of IDN-6556 (3-[2-(2-tert-butyl-phenylaminooxalyl)-amino]-propionylamino]-4-oxo-5-(2,3,5,6-tetrafluoro-phenoxy)-pentanoic acid): a liver-targeted caspase inhibitor. J Pharmacol Exp Ther 2004;309(2):634–40.
28. Canbay A, Feldstein A, Baskin-Bey E, et al. The caspase inhibitor IDN-6556 attenuates hepatic injury and fibrosis in the bile duct ligated mouse. J Pharmacol Exp Ther 2004;308(3):1191–6.
29. Pockros PJ, Schiff ER, Shiffman ML, et al. Oral IDN-6556, an antiapoptotic caspase inhibitor, lowers aminotransferases in patients with chronic hepatitis C. Hepatology 2007;46(2):324–9.
30. Available at: ClinicalTrials.gov. Identifier: NCT00725803. Accessed March 6, 2009.

Antisense Inhibitors, Ribozymes, and siRNAs

Alexander J.V. Thompson, MD, PhD, Keyur Patel, MD*

KEYWORDS

• Chronic hepatitis C • Antisense • Oligonucleotide • Ribozyme
• siRNA • shRNA • RNA interference

The current standard of care for the treatment of patients with chronic hepatitis C virus (HCV) infection is expensive, poorly tolerated, and effective in only 50% of eligible patients. Alternative therapies are needed, particularly for patients with genotype 1 infection. Although the ongoing development of small molecule protease and polymerase inhibitors represents a significant therapeutic advance, a significant minority of patients may remain refractory.[1–3]

Oligonucleotide (ON)-based therapies have great potential for the treatment of RNA viruses such as HCV. They include antisense oligonucleotides (ASONs) and their derivatives (peptide nucleic acids, locked nucleic acids, and morpholinos ONs), RNAi, ribozymes and aptamers. ON-based approaches depend on the Watson-Crick base pairing of oligonucleotides to their corresponding mRNA target. This leads to post-transcriptional gene silencing through mRNA cleavage or translational inhibition. Much progress has been made in the application of this technology to the treatment of HCV over the past decade, with inhibition of viral replication demonstrated in vitro. However, successful clinical translation has been limited by a lack of efficient delivery systems, safety concerns, and the specter of antiviral resistance.

HCV MOLECULAR BIOLOGY

The hepatitis C virus is a member of the Flaviviridae family, and has a positive-sense ssRNA genome that functions as mRNA for the viral polyprotein and the template for reverse transcription (**Fig. 1**). In theory, it is an attractive target for oligonucleotide therapy, which might be designed to target multiple regions in the viral sequence. Unfortunately, HCV shows remarkable sequence variation, which is challenging for ON drug design. HCV is divided into 6 major genotypes on the basis of nucleotide

This work has been supported by the IMS Overseas Travelling Fellowship (Royal Australasian College of Physicians) and a Postdoctoral Overseas Based Biomedical Fellowship (National Health and Medical Research Council of Australia).
Division of Gastroenterology/Hepatology, Duke Clinical Research Institute, Duke University, PO Box 17969, Durham, NC 27715, USA
* Corresponding author.
E-mail address: keyur.patel@duke.edu (K. Patel).

Clin Liver Dis 13 (2009) 375–390
doi:10.1016/j.cld.2009.05.003

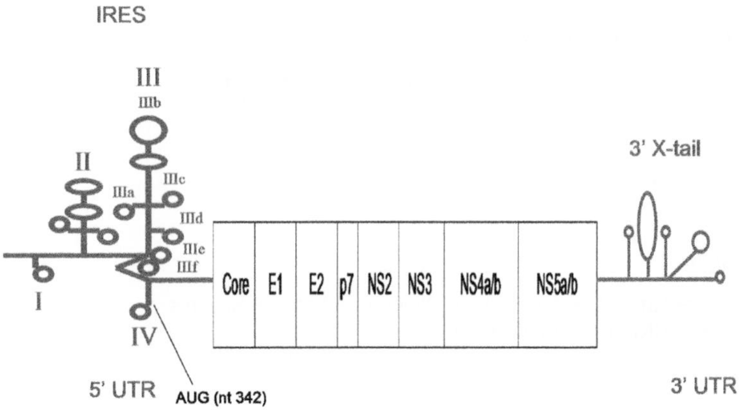

Fig. 1. DICER is an endoribonuclease in the RNase III family that generates 19 to 23 nt dsRNA products (siRNA) from long dsRNA or shRNA. These are directed to the RISC complex, which removes the sense strand and pairs the antisense strand with a complementary region of "target" mRNA (matched perfectly to the "seed" region of antisense strand, nt 2–7 from the 5′ end). RISC then directs the cleavage of the target mRNA at a site between nt 10 and 11 relative to the 5′ end of the antisense strand. The cleaved 5′ and 3′ mRNA fragments are degraded by cellular nucleases. Alternatively, RISC may direct translational arrest, particularly in the setting of a partially complementary siRNA sequence. Long dsRNA (>30 nt length) may also trigger a type 1 IFN response, which leads to global inhibition of protein translation. siRNA, small inhibitory RNA; dsRNA, double-stranded RNA; shRNA, short hairpin RNA; RISC, RNA-induced silencing complex; TLR3, Toll-like receptor 3; RIG-I, retinoic acid inducible gene I; MDA-5, melanoma differentiation-associated gene-5; IFN, interferon; OAS, oligoadenylate synthetase; PKR, RNA-dependent protein kinase; P, phosphate; eIF-2α, eukaryotic translation initiation factor-2α.

(nt) sequence divergence of at least 30%.[4] The genotype groups are divided into at least 52 subtypes defined by sequence divergence of 20% to 25%. In addition, HCV exists within its host as a quasispecies, a pool of genetically distinct but closely related variants. This heterogeneity is driven by the error-prone HCV RNA polymerase, which has an error rate in the order of 10^{-3} to 10^{-5} mutations per nt per genomic replication.[5–7] This is an important issue for the design of effective ON-based therapy for HCV, which relies on precise sequence complementarity. Fortunately, there are highly conserved regions within the HCV genome that have been identified. These sequences include regions of the internal ribosomal entry site (IRES) of the 5′ untranslated region (UTR), in particular domain IIId, which contains the 40S ribosomal subunit binding site, and domain IV, which contains the AUG translational initiation site. The IIId domain contains a sequence that seems to be invariant across all genotypes described.[8–11] Other potential targets include the X-tail of the 3′ UTR, and short sequences of the core protein and the NS5B polymerase.[12]

Beyond sequence conservation, a second consideration is that the RNA target must be accessible to ONs. The secondary structure of mRNA target sites has been reported to strongly influence RNAi activity.[13–15] To allow for this, the most common approach to drug design involves database mining coupled with computer programs that predict RNA secondary structures. Unfortunately predicting the secondary structure of de novo HCV RNA has proven difficult, and potential targets must be verified experimentally.[16] The development of the genotype 1 replicon system, and more recently the JFH-1 genotype 2a infectious clone, has greatly facilitated this screening process (with the caveat that these models are genotype specific).

ANTISENSE OLIGONUCLEOTIDES

Antisense oligonucleotides (ASONs) are short single-stranded segments of DNA or RNA, typically 12 to 26 bases in length. They act by binding to a complementary sequence of mRNA and RNA, and blocking gene expression (**Fig. 2**), which may occur through 1 of 2 major mechanisms: RNase H–dependent cleavage of target RNA or RNase H–independent steric blockade of RNA processing. Although RNase H–dependent gene silencing may confer some advantages compared with steric blockade, it may be less suitable for targeting HCV. The life cycle of HCV occurs entirely within the cytoplasm, whereas RNase H principally resides in the nucleus. Therefore, ASONs acting by steric blockade may be more effective. The mechanism of action is largely determined by the chemical structure of the ASON. Numerous chemical modifications have been introduced into the nucleotide backbone to improve base pair affinity, target specificity, biologic stability, and reduce toxicity.

Phosphorothioate oligonucleotides are the most common compounds to have progressed to clinical studies (eg, ISIS 14803, ISIS Pharmaceuticals, Carlsbad, CA, discussed later). Phosphorothioates efficiently recruit and activate endogenous RNase H.[17] Phosphorothioate modification also offers the benefits of nuclease resistance and high solubility, without major changes in the ability to hybridize to target RNA.[18] Unfortunately, phosphorothioate ONs are negatively charged and have a tendency to nonspecifically bind serum proteins, including thrombin. Coagulation defects

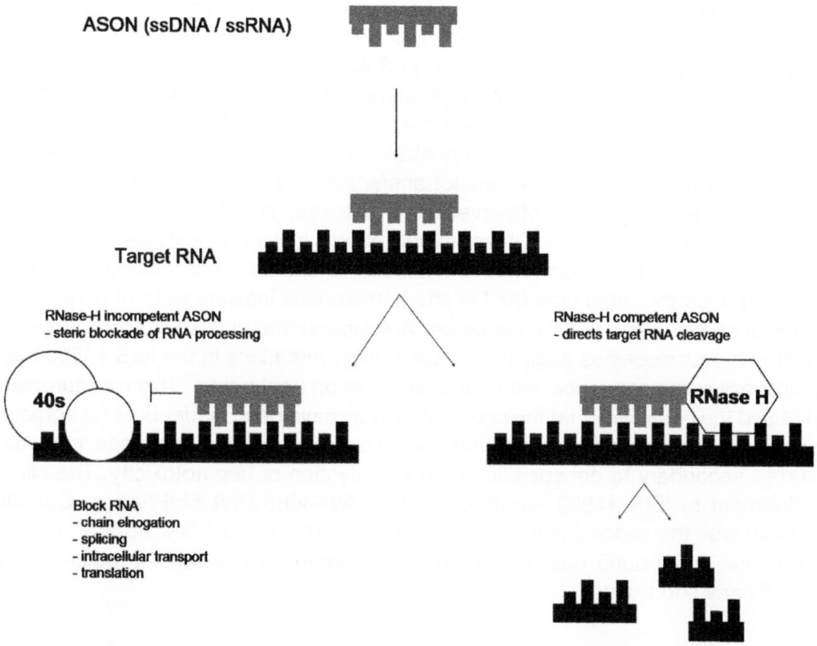

Fig. 2. The HCV genome is a positive-sense ssRNA molecule. It contains one 9.6 kb open reading frame flanked by 2 highly conserved untranslated regions (UTR) (highlighted in red). The open reading frame encodes the HCV polyprotein precursor, which is co- and post-translationally processed to yield 10 mature proteins (3 structural [core, E1, and E2] and nonstructural [NS; p7, NS2, NS3, NS4a, NS4b, NS5a and NS5b]). The position of the polyprotein start codon within domain IV of the IRES is noted. IRES, internal ribosomal entry site.

have been reported.[19,20] ASONs have also been associated with nonspecific immunostimulatory effects on B cells, attributed to CpG motifs within the nucleotide sequence.[21] CpG motifs are now recognized to be a ligand for Toll-like receptor 9 (TLR9), a potent activator of immune cells.[22]

Compounds with alternative nucleotide backbones have been developed to minimize toxicity. N3′ to P5′ phosphoroamidates are an example.[23] These compounds do not activate RNase H, but provide steric blockade of protein translation. Chimeric ONs, containing a mixture of natural and modified nucleotides that preserve RNase H–inducing affinity, represent another strategy that takes advantage of both antisense pathways, while maintaining the improved binding, pharmacokinetic, and toxicity profiles.[24] More recently, several other highly modified oligonucleotides that aim to improve compound stability and half-life have emerged, including locked nucleic acids (LNAs), peptide nucleic acids (PNAs) and morpholino compounds.

The most common targets of anti-HCV ASON design have been located within the highly conserved regions of the 5′ UTR IRES, including the IIId loop, the pyrimidine rich tract in domain II and the AUG codon in domain IV.[25,26] Other targets have included conserved segments within the 3′ X-tail, the core protein coding region, and the NS3 coding sequence.[25,26] Although multiple drug candidates have demonstrated efficacy in preclinical evaluation, only 2 compounds have progressed to clinical trials.

ISIS 14803 (Isis Pharmaceuticals, Carlsbad, CA, USA) was the first ASON to enter clinical trials for the treatment of chronic HCV infection. ISIS 14803 is a 20-unit phosphorothioate oligodeoxynucleotide designed to be complementary to the HCV 5′ UTR at nt 330 to 349, which includes the AUG start codon for HCV polyprotein translation. ISIS 14803 inhibited HCV replication and protein expression in cell culture and mouse models by directing RNA cleavage through RNase H.[27,28] A phase I dose escalation study was performed in patients with genotype 1 chronic hepatitis C (CHC), most of whom were previous interferon (IFN)-nonresponders.[20] Unfortunately, reduction in serum HCV RNA of >1 $\log_{10}$ IU/mL was observed in only 3/28 patients. Furthermore, reversible, asymptomatic alanine aminotransferase (ALT) flares (9–18 times the upper limit of normal [ULN]) were observed in 5 patients, including all 3 patients who achieved a virologic response. Other adverse effects included local injection site reactions from subcutaneous administration, headache, and transient prolongation of activated partial prothrombin time (APTT) after intravenous infusion without hemorrhagic complications or other clinical sequelae. A substudy that investigated HCV genetic evolution by quasispecies analysis did not identify mutations in the ISIS 14803 target site or surrounding sequence, either at baseline or on treatment.[29] This was surprising, and raised the possibility that the doses used may have been inadequate for achieving a specific antisense effect, and that the observed virologic response may have occurred secondary to nonspecific immune activation or hepatotoxicity. The clinical development of ISIS 14803 has been halted. AVI-4065 (AVI BioPharma, Corvallis, OR, USA) was the second antisense inhibitor to enter clinical trials. Further development of this compound has also been halted, after early phase II studies did not meet efficacy end points.

OTHER MODIFIED OLIGONUCLEOTIDES

Other oligonucleotide candidates are characterized by more radical modifications that aim to improve stability. These include the PNAs, morpholino compounds, and LNAs, which have been developed to increase target affinity and minimize nuclease sensitivity and toxicity. All function through steric inhibition of RNA translation and are RNase H independent.

Peptide nucleic acids are nucleic acid analogs consisting of natural nucleoside bases on a pseudopeptide backbone.[30] Compared with phosphorothioate ONs, PNAs have improved selectivity and affinity to target DNA or RNA, lower affinity to proteins, and are highly resistant to nuclease and peptidase degradation.[31] PNAs targeting the 5′ UTR have been shown to have an antiviral effect in vitro.[32,33] One drawback of PNAs is their chemical neutrality and poor solubility, resulting in limited cellular uptake and difficulties with incorporation into carrier molecules. The recent demonstration of short PNAs (<17-mer) with anti-HCV activity may facilitate the design of agents suitable for therapeutic administration.[33]

Morpholino molecules are a third generation ASON that contain nucleic acid bases bound to morpholine rings instead of deoxyribose rings, linked by phosphorodiamidate groups instead of phosphates.[34] The morpholino structure affords excellent RNA binding affinity, water solubility, and nuclease resistance. Like PNAs, they are neutral molecules, increasing the challenges of effective delivery to the intracellular compartment. Morpholino ONs targeting the HCV IRES have demonstrated efficacy in vitro.[35,36]

Locked nucleic acid nucleotides contain a bridging methylene carbon between the 2′ and 4′ positions of the ribose ring.[32,37] This linkage constrains ("locks") the conformation of the ribose ring and preorganizes the LNA base for hybridization to mRNA, enhancing the binding affinity for complementary sequence. LNA ONs have been reported to have potent biologic activity in vivo; anti-HCV activity has been reported in vitro.[32] More recently, LNAs have been reported to cause hepatotoxicity in mouse models.[38] This issue will need to be addressed before human studies can be considered.

RIBOZYMES

Ribozymes are catalytic RNAs, originally described in the protozoa *Tetrahymena thermophilia*.[39–41] Naturally occurring ribozymes are self-splicing, but chemical modifications have allowed ribozymes that cleave complementary target RNA to be engineered (**Fig. 3**). Thus, ribozymes retain the target specificity of ASON technology without the requirement for RNase H–mediated cleavage. In theory, this would be of benefit as HCV replicates within the cytoplasm, where little RNase H is found. However, one difficulty in ribozyme design is that catalytic activity is highly structure-dependent, thus limiting the ability to improve pharmacokinetics, efficacy, or toxicity by chemical modulation. The chemical structure of the more common "hammerhead" ribozyme consists of 2 short HCV annealing arms flanking a catalytic core (the annealing arms are designed to recognize the selected HCV target sequence). Following target cleavage, the ribozyme is released and recycled for continued rounds of cleavage. Anti-HCV ribozymes designed to target conserved regions of the HCV genome have been effective in laboratory models.[42–48]

Heptazyme (Ribozyme Pharmaceuticals, Boulder, CO, USA) was the first oligonucleotide-based therapy to enter phase II clinical development for HCV infection. Heptazyme, a 33-nt nuclease-stabilized ribozyme directed against the 5′ UTR IRES, demonstrated potent anti-HCV activity in vitro.[48–50] In phase I studies, Heptazyme was well tolerated, and early phase II testing demonstrated biologically meaningful reductions in serum HCV RNA levels in 10% of patients.[51] Unfortunately, phase II clinical development was halted after the occurrence of blindness in a test animal. No ribozymes are currently in clinical development.

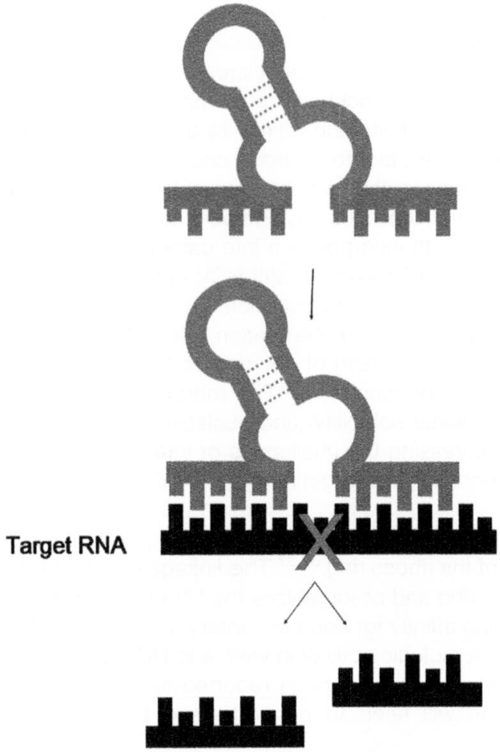

Fig. 3. The mechanism of action of antisense oligonucleotides.

DEOXYRIBOZYMES

Deoxyribozymes (Dz) are single-stranded DNA molecules that cleave homologous RNA targets.[52] They are typically 30 to 40 nt in length, and consist of a central catalytic core flanked by 2 short ASON annealing arms. They combine features of ASONs and ribozymes, but have advantages over both. Dz can be engineered to cleave virtually any large RNA target. They are more resistant to nuclease degradation following chemical modification, are less expensive to synthesize, and have greater catalytic efficiency than ribozymes. Dz targeting the IRES and core regions have been used to inhibit HCV replication in vitro.[53–55]

RNA INTERFERENCE

RNAi is an emerging therapeutic modality for the silencing of gene expression. A conserved evolutionary pathway, RNAi was first recognized in 1998 as the biologic response to exogenous double-stranded RNA (dsRNA) in *Caenorhabditis elegans*.[56] It is based on the complementarity of "short" dsRNA sequences, leading to target-specific silencing of gene expression. In contrast, "long" dsRNA sequences trigger the type 1 IFN response and nonspecific inhibition of protein translation. It is the length of the dsRNA sequence that is critical in determining the cellular response.

"Long" dsRNA sequences, greater than 30 nt in length, are common structural components of viral replicative intermediates, including HCV. Long dsRNA activates the pattern recognition receptors TLR3, RIG-I, or MDA-5;[57] downstream signaling by way of IRF-3 induces type 1 IFNs (IFNβ) and global inhibition of cellular protein translation (see **Fig. 4**). IFN has pleiotropic cellular effects and also induces genes that lead to apoptosis, increased major histocompatibility complex (MHC) class I expression (helping natural killer [NK] cells to distinguish viral-infected targets), and signals that activate the antiviral response of neighboring cells, impeding the propagation of viral infection.

In mammalian cells, long dsRNAs are also cleaved into "short" dsRNA segments by the cytoplasmic enzyme DICER (**Fig. 4**).[58] The 21 to 23 nt dsRNA products (siRNA) are then directed to the RNA-induced silencing complex (RISC) complex, which directs sequence-specific mRNA cleavage (**Fig. 4**)[59,60] gene silencing. It is this process of sequence-specific gene silencing that is termed RNA inhibition, or RNAi.

Short interfering RNA (siRNA)-induced gene suppression is usually transient. Plasmidvector systems containing short hairpin RNA (shRNA) sequences have been developed as a mechanism for continuous delivery of RNA interference (RNAi). shRNA are short sequences of RNA that contain a tight hairpin turn, and are processed intracellularly by DICER into siRNA (**Fig. 4**). An example of a viral delivery system is the family of adeno-associated viruses (AAV). AAV form episomal DNA molecules, from which shRNA can be continuously expressed under the control of ubiquitous promoters such as U6. Furthermore, this vector may be passed onto daughter cells, allowing gene silencing to be inherited. Despite efficacy in vitro, concerns persist about the clinical safety of viral vectors (discussed later).

Direct delivery to a cell of siRNA fragments (<30 nt long) avoids the nonspecific IFN response while retaining the target-specific RNAi activity.[61] RNAi has proven a powerful scientific tool, allowing gene "knockout" experiments that were previously limited to the domain of small animal model systems to be performed on almost any cell type. There is considerable therapeutic potential for siRNA targeting of oncogenes and infectious organisms. The potent anti-HCV efficacy of RNAi has been demonstrated in replicon cell culture models[62] and transgenic mouse models,[63–69] whereby up to

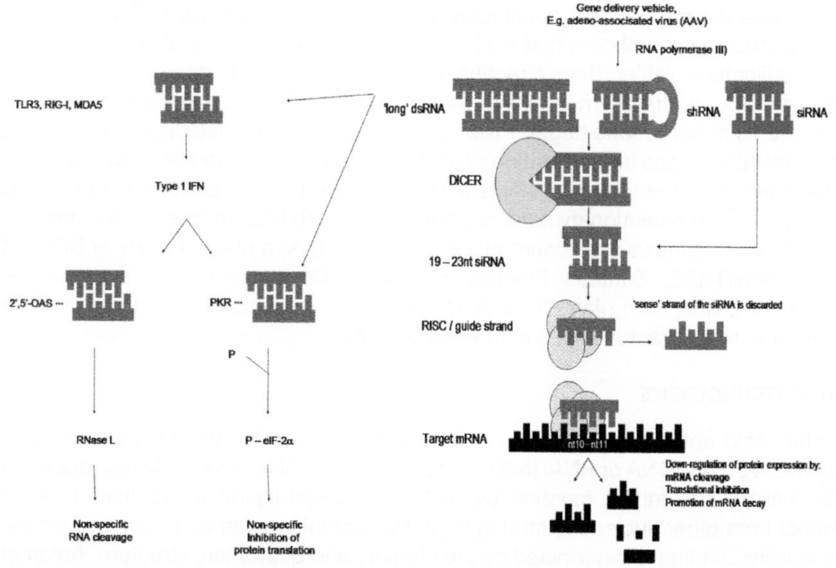

Fig. 4. Anti-HCV ribozymes consists of 2 short HCV annealing arms flanking a catalytic core, which cleaves the target sequence.

80-fold reductions in HCV RNA have been demonstrated. Other studies using the HCV replicon system have shown clearance of replication-competent HCV RNA from more that 98% of cells following siRNA delivery.[70,71] Early RNAi designs targeted the HCV NS5B polymerase;[63] more recent candidates have targeted conserved regions of the genome, most commonly the 5′ UTR IRES but also RNA segments in the 3′ UTR, core, E2, NS3, and NS4B.

Several pharmaceutical companies are investigating the development of anti-HCV RNAi candidates, including TT-033 (Tacere Therapeutics, San Jose, CA). TT-033 employs a multi-targeted approach using 3 shRNA complementary to sequences in the 5′ UTR and the NS5B. A second candidate is SIRNA-034 (Merck, Whitehouse Station, NJ, USA). However, none have yet entered clinical development, with ongoing concerns regarding effective delivery and the risk of off-target effects.

MICRORNA

MicroRNAs (miRNA) are endogenous, short (~22 nt), noncoding RNAs, which constitute a naturally occurring pathway of post-transcriptional gene regulation by RNAi. Although miRNA and siRNA use the same cellular machinery, they are distinguished by their mode of biogenesis (shRNA are mimics of pre-miRNA) (**Fig. 5**).[72] It has recently been shown that homology of only the "seed region" (nt 2–7 from the miRNA 5′ end) is required, increasing the potential/risk for off-target silencing of partially complementary genes.[73] It is believed that the human genome encodes at least 800 miRNA,[74] some of which are ubiquitous, but others seem highly tissue-specific. miRNA have been implicated in the regulation of genes involved in cell growth and differentiation, apoptosis and oncogenesis, and have been identified more recently as putative IFN-stimulated genes (ISGs), perhaps contributing to the antiviral effect of type 1 IFN.[75] Indeed, IFNβ-inducible cellular miRNAs have been identified with complementary sequence to the HCV genome, which could inhibit HCV replication in vitro (miR-196, miR-296, miR-351, miR-451 and miR-448).[76–80]

miR-122 has been identified as a permissive factor for HCV replication. miR-122 is a liver-specific miRNA that constitutes 70% of total hepatocyte miRNA.[77] Experimental studies have shown that miR-122 interacts with the HCV 5′ UTR to facilitate viral replication, rather than directing the silencing of viral gene expression.[81,82] Although the underlying mechanism remains unclear, this has generated interest in miR-122 as a therapeutic target. Proof-of-concept has been established in primates, whereby intravenous administration of a locked nucleic acid–modified oligonucleotide (LNA-antimir) was observed to efficiently silence miR-122 expression without obvious toxicity.[83–85] On a cautionary note, suppression of miR-122 has been associated with hepatocarcinogenesis in a rodent model.[86] Despite this, a phase I study of SPC3649 (LNA-antimiR-122, Santaris Pharma, Hørsholm, Denmark) in healthy volunteers has commenced, with plans for a phase II study in patients with CHC (http://www.seventure.fr/fileup/actualite/seventureActu38.pdf).

OTHER TECHNOLOGIES

Nucleic acid aptamers (derived from the Latin *aptus*, to fit) are short sequences of oligonucleotides (DNA or RNA) that bind to a protein or RNA target with high specificity and affinity, and inhibit function by restricting target-ligand interaction. They are distinct from other nucleotide strategies, in that complementarity is not a requirement for activity; binding is determined by their tertiary and quaternary structure. Aptamers are generated by the SELEX (Systematic Evolution of Ligands by Selective Enrichment) process, involving high throughput screening of DNA libraries and subsequent

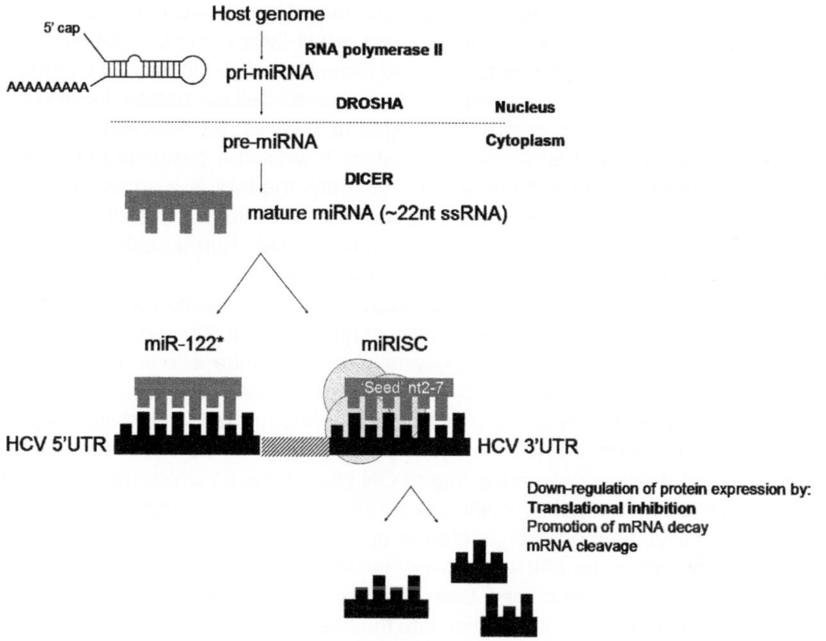

Fig. 5. MicroRNAs (miRNA) arise from noncoding intergenic or intronic regions, as transcripts that form stem-loop structures called pri-miRNA. Pri-miRNA are processed first in the nucleus, by DROSHA, before exportin-5-mediated transport to the cytoplasm as a 65 to 75 nt pre-miRNA, which is further processed by DICER to mature miRNA. Cytoplasmic miRNA is assembled into the RISC (miRISC), the effector of RNAi. RISC-bound miRNAs then guide the recognition of complementary regions within the 3′ UTR of the target mRNA. Target recognition requires homology of only nt 2 to 7 from the miRNA 5′ end (the "seed" region); partial homology to the remaining sequence is tolerated. miRNA directed cleavage of target mRNA is unusual; inhibition of translation is more common. miR-122 has a unique relationship with the 5′ UTR of the HCV genome (see text).

amplification, cloning, and sequencing.[87,88] Aptamers therefore combine the advantages of therapeutic antibodies (equivalent binding specificity, affinity) with those of small molecule therapeutics (ease of chemical synthesis, amenable to nucleotide modifications, and nonimmunogenic). Aptamers targeting the HCV NS5B polymerase, NS3 protease, 5′ UTR/IRES and 3′ UTR have been used in vitro to inhibit HCV enzyme function or HCV protein translation, respectively.[89–97] Clinical development has not yet been reported.

CHALLENGES

Despite the in vitro demonstration of efficacy of oligonucleotide-based therapies, several significant challenges will need to be overcome before further clinical development in HCV infection is possible. Important issues include (1) effective delivery to the target organ/cell, (2) safety (off-target effects/IFN induction/toxicity), and (3) viral resistance.

Delivery

The effective delivery of antisense therapies to their intended site of action remains a significant obstacle for this emerging therapeutic field. Oligonucleotides are not bioavailable, and must be administered parenterally. Unmodified, "naked" ONs are degraded rapidly by nucleases, resulting in short half-lives in the circulation. Due to the hydrophobic nature of the membrane lipid bilayer, passive diffusion of oligonucleotides across intact cell membranes is not observed. Cellular uptake likely occurs through endocytosis. This presents challenges at 2 levels: the vascular endothelial barrier and the target cell membrane. In addition, it would be desirable to target ON specifically to the organ/cell of interest. Fortunately, the liver is a somewhat "privileged" target, due to the fenestrated nature of the sinusoidal epithelium. However, accumulation of ONs in nonparenchymal cells, particularly Kupffer cells, is an issue, and hepatocyte-specific delivery systems are required.

Antisense delivery in vitro is typically achieved through transfection or hyperdynamic injection, neither of which is suitable for clinical development. One solution is the use of supramolecular nanocarriers (eg, liposomes). A single intravenous dose of a liposomal formulation of ApoB-specific siRNA has recently been shown to successfully silence gene expression in a primate model.[98] Although mild hepatotoxicity was observed at high doses, the technology is promising. Other potential strategies for chemical-based delivery include the use of ON conjugates (in which the ON is complexed to a ligand that targets specific cell surface receptors or enhances transmembrane permeability), antibody conjugates or aptamer-siRNA chimeras. Although viral vectors have proved to be efficient delivery systems in cell culture and small animal models, clinical development has been hindered by concerns about the consequences of random retroviral integration into the host genome, as well as the induction of toxic immune responses.[99]

Safety

Several safety concerns persist regarding the clinical use of antisense and RNAi therapies. The risk of off-target gene silencing (whereby the target sequence is present in multiple mRNAs),[73,100–103] the risk of saturating the endogenous miRNA pathway (recently shown to cause hepatotoxicity in mice[104]), and the risk of unintended IFN induction by way of dsRNA-TLR3[105,106] or ssRNA-TLR7/8[107] stimulation (although IFN induction may be beneficial for anti-HCV therapy) have been described. Furthermore, there are only limited toxicity data in primates (the safety species of choice for maximizing the detection of off-target effects), and almost no data in humans, indicating that unsuspected or idiosyncratic toxicities have yet be uncovered.

Resistance

The sequence specificity of antisense ON or RNAi, one of the technology's most attractive properties, is a double-edged sword. Although this allows the HCV RNA genome to be targeted at the nucleotide level, it also means that substitutions of only 1 or 2 nucleotides confer resistance. Given the high error rate of the HCV RNA polymerase, it is not surprising that in vitro resistance has already been reported.[108,109] Experimental approaches that have been designed to limit the emergence of resistance include targeting highly conserved regions of the genome, using combination treatment with several agents targeting different sites in the genome,[108,110] and the more novel long-hairpin RNA.[15]

Finally, certain viruses have evolved mechanisms for suppressing RNAi. For example, vaccinia virus E3L, influenza NS1[111] and adenovirus noncoding VA1 RNA[112] have been shown to suppress siRNA machinery. HIV tat protein inhibits RNAi by subverting DICER processing in vitro.[113] Although not yet demonstrated for HCV, there are little data available and further investigation is warranted. Identification of similar strategies for suppression of siRNA activity would further limit therapeutic application.

SUMMARY

Antisense and siRNA oligonucleotides remain invaluable laboratory tools, and have great potential for therapeutic application. Potent antiviral effects against HCV have been demonstrated in vitro. However, safe and effective delivery to the hepatocyte has not yet been achieved in vivo. Furthermore, HCV presents particular difficulties for molecular technologies reliant on precise sequence complementarity, due to its remarkable sequence diversity and error-prone replication. However, RNAi research, basic and translational, is progressing rapidly, and it is hoped that with greater insight into the endogenous RNAi pathways, and development of novel delivery methods, clinical application of this technology to HCV infection will be possible in the not-too-distant future.

REFERENCES

1. McHutchison JG, Everson GT, Gordon SC, et al. PROVE1: results from a phase 2 study of telaprevir with peginterferon alfa-2a and ribavirin in treatment-naive subjects with hepatitis C [abstract (4)]. J Hepatol 2008;48:S4.
2. Zeuzem S, Hezode C, Ferenci P, et al. Telaprevir in combination with peginterferon-alfa-2a with or without ribavirin in the treatment of chronic hepatitis C: final results of the PROVE2 study [abstract (243)]. Hepatology 2008;48:418A.
3. Kwo P, Lawitz EJ, McCone J, et al. HCV SPRINT-1: boceprevir plus peginterferon alfa-2b/ribavirin for treatment of genotype 1 chronic hepatitis C in previously untreated patients [abstract]. Hepatology 2008;48:1027A.
4. Penin F, Dubuisson J, Rey FA, et al. Structural biology of hepatitis C virus. Hepatology 2004;39:5–19.
5. Bartenschlager R, Lohmann V. Replication of hepatitis C virus. J Gen Virol 2000; 81:1631–48.
6. Bukh J, Miller RH, Purcell RH. Genetic heterogeneity of hepatitis C virus: quasispecies and genotypes. Semin Liver Dis 1995;15:41–63.
7. Duffy S, Shackelton LA, Holmes EC. Rates of evolutionary change in viruses: patterns and determinants. Nat Rev Genet 2008;9:267–76.
8. Bukh J, Purcell RH, Miller RH. Sequence analysis of the 5′ noncoding region of hepatitis C virus. Proc Natl Acad Sci U S A 1992;89:4942–6.
9. Kieft JS, Zhou K, Jubin R, et al. The hepatitis C virus internal ribosome entry site adopts an ion-dependent tertiary fold. J Mol Biol 1999;292:513–29.
10. Martinand-Mari C, Lebleu B, Robbins I. Oligonucleotide-based strategies to inhibit human hepatitis C virus. Oligonucleotides 2003;13:539–48.
11. Dasgupta A, Das S, Izumi R, et al. Targeting internal ribosome entry site (IRES)-mediated translation to block hepatitis C and other RNA viruses. FEMS Microbiol Lett 2004;234:189–99.
12. Blight KJ, Kolykhalov AA, Rice CM. Efficient initiation of HCV RNA replication in cell culture. Science 2000;290:1972–4.
13. Brown KM, Chu CY, Rana TM. Target accessibility dictates the potency of human RISC. Nat Struct Mol Biol 2005;12:469–70.
14. Overhoff M, Alken M, Far RK, et al. Local RNA target structure influences siRNA efficacy: a systematic global analysis. J Mol Biol 2005;348:871–81.

15. Watanabe T, Sudoh M, Miyagishi M, et al. Intracellular-diced dsRNA has enhanced efficacy for silencing HCV RNA and overcomes variation in the viral genotype. Gene Ther 2006;13:883–92.
16. Sohail M, Southern EM. Selecting optimal antisense reagents. Adv Drug Deliv Rev 2000;44:23–34.
17. Zamaratski E, Pradeepkumar PI, Chattopadhyaya J. A critical survey of the structure-function of the antisense oligo/RNA heteroduplex as substrate for RNase H. J Biochem Biophys Methods 2001;48:189–208.
18. Kurreck J. Antisense technologies. Improvement through novel chemical modifications. Eur J Biochem 2003;270:1628–44.
19. Henry SP, Novotny W, Leeds J, et al. Inhibition of coagulation by a phosphorothioate oligonucleotide. Antisense Nucleic Acid Drug Dev 1997;7:503–10.
20. McHutchison JG, Patel K, Pockros P, et al. A phase I trial of an antisense inhibitor of hepatitis C virus (ISIS 14803), administered to chronic hepatitis C patients. J Hepatol 2006;44:88–96.
21. Liang H, Nishioka Y, Reich CF, et al. Activation of human B cells by phosphorothioate oligodeoxynucleotides. J Clin Invest 1996;98:1119–29.
22. Hemmi H, Takeuchi O, Kawai T, et al. A Toll-like receptor recognizes bacterial DNA. Nature 2000;408:740–5.
23. Gryaznov S, Skorski T, Cucco C, et al. Oligonucleotide N3′→P5′ phosphoramidates as antisense agents. Nucleic Acids Res 1996;24:1508–14.
24. Agrawal S. Importance of nucleotide sequence and chemical modifications of antisense oligonucleotides. Biochim Biophys Acta 1999;1489:53–68.
25. Trepanier JB, Tanner JE, Alfieri C. Oligonucleotide-based therapeutic options against hepatitis C virus infection. Antivir Ther 2006;11:273–87.
26. Watanabe T, Umehara T, Kohara M. Therapeutic application of RNA interference for hepatitis C virus. Adv Drug Deliv Rev 2007;59:1263–76.
27. Hanecak R, Brown-Driver V, Fox MC, et al. Antisense oligonucleotide inhibition of hepatitis C virus gene expression in transformed hepatocytes. J Virol 1996;70:5203–12.
28. Zhang H, Hanecak R, Brown-Driver V, et al. Antisense oligonucleotide inhibition of hepatitis C virus (HCV) gene expression in livers of mice infected with an HCV-vaccinia virus recombinant. Antimicrobial Agents Chemother 1999;43:347–53.
29. Soler M, McHutchison JG, Kwoh TJ, et al. Virological effects of ISIS 14803, an antisense oligonucleotide inhibitor of hepatitis C virus (HCV) internal ribosome entry site (IRES), on HCV IRES in chronic hepatitis C patients and examination of the potential role of primary and secondary HCV resistance in the outcome of treatment. Antivir Ther 2004;9:953–68.
30. Nielsen PE, Egholm M, Berg RH, et al. Sequence-selective recognition of DNA by strand displacement with a thymine-substituted polyamide. Science 1991;254:1497–500.
31. Demidov VV, Potaman VN, Frank-Kamenetskii MD, et al. Stability of peptide nucleic acids in human serum and cellular extracts. Biochem Pharmacol 1994;48:1310–3.
32. Nulf CJ, Corey D. Intracellular inhibition of hepatitis C virus (HCV) internal ribosomal entry site (IRES)-dependent translation by peptide nucleic acids (PNAs) and locked nucleic acids (LNAs). Nucleic Acids Res 2004;32:3792–8.
33. Alotte C, Martin A, Caldarelli SA, et al. Short peptide nucleic acids (PNA) inhibit hepatitis C virus internal ribosome entry site (IRES) dependent translation in vitro. Antiviral Res 2008;80:280–7.
34. Summerton J, Weller D. Morpholino antisense oligomers: design, preparation, and properties. Antisense Nucleic Acid Drug Dev 1997;7:187–95.

35. McCaffrey AP, Meuse L, Karimi M, et al. A potent and specific morpholino antisense inhibitor of hepatitis C translation in mice. Hepatology 2003;38:503–8.
36. Jubin R, Vantuno NE, Kieft JS, et al. Hepatitis C virus internal ribosome entry site (IRES) stem loop IIId contains a phylogenetically conserved GGG triplet essential for translation and IRES folding. J Virol 2000;74:10430–7.
37. Corey DR. Chemical modification: the key to clinical application of RNA interference? J Clin Invest 2007;117:3615–22.
38. Swayze EE, Siwkowski AM, Wancewicz EV, et al. Antisense oligonucleotides containing locked nucleic acid improve potency but cause significant hepatotoxicity in animals. Nucleic Acids Res 2007;35:687–700.
39. Guerrier-Takada C, Gardiner K, Marsh T, et al. The RNA moiety of ribonuclease P is the catalytic subunit of the enzyme. Cell 1983;35:849–57.
40. Cech TR, Zaug AJ, Grabowski PJ. In vitro splicing of the ribosomal RNA precursor of tetrahymena: involvement of a guanosine nucleotide in the excision of the intervening sequence. Cell 1981;27:487–96.
41. Shippy R, Lockner R, Farnsworth M, et al. The hairpin ribozyme. Discovery, mechanism, and development for gene therapy. Mol Biotechnol 1999;12:117–29.
42. Gonzalez-Carmona MA, Schussler S, Serwe M, et al. Hammerhead ribozymes with cleavage site specificity for NUH and NCH display significant anti-hepatitis C viral effect in vitro and in recombinant HepG2 and CCL13 cells. J Hepatol 2006;44:1017–25.
43. Lieber A, He CY, Polyak SJ, et al. Elimination of hepatitis C virus RNA in infected human hepatocytes by adenovirus-mediated expression of ribozymes. J Virol 1996;70:8782–91.
44. Sabariegos R, Nadal A, Beguiristain N, et al. Catalytic RNase P RNA from *Synechocystis* sp. cleaves the hepatitis C virus RNA near the AUG start codon. FEBS Lett 2004;577:517–22.
45. Sakamoto N, Wu CH, Wu GY. Intracellular cleavage of hepatitis C virus RNA and inhibition of viral protein translation by hammerhead ribozymes. J Clin Invest 1996;98:2720–8.
46. Welch PJ, Tritz R, Yei S, et al. A potential therapeutic application of hairpin ribozymes: in vitro and in vivo studies of gene therapy for hepatitis C virus infection. Gene Ther 1996;3:994–1001.
47. Nadal A, Robertson HD, Guardia J, et al. Characterization of the structure and variability of an internal region of hepatitis C virus RNA for M1 RNA guide sequence ribozyme targeting. J Gen Virol 2003;84:1545–8.
48. Macejak DG, Jensen KL, Jamison SF, et al. Inhibition of hepatitis C virus (HCV)-RNA-dependent translation and replication of a chimeric HCV poliovirus using synthetic stabilized ribozymes. Hepatology 2000;31:769–76.
49. Usman N, Blatt LM. Nuclease-resistant synthetic ribozymes: developing a new class of therapeutics. J Clin Invest 2000;106:1197–202.
50. Brown-Augsburger P, Yue XM, Lockridge JA, et al. Development and validation of a sensitive, specific, and rapid hybridization-ELISA assay for determination of concentrations of a ribozyme in biological matrices. J Pharm Biomed Anal 2004;34:129–39.
51. Tong MJ, Schiff E, Jensen D, et al. Preliminary analysis of a phase II study of heptazyme, a nuclease resistant ribozyme targeting hepatitis C virus (HCV) RNA [abstract (788)]. Hepatology 2002;36(4), Part 2:360A.
52. Santoro SW, Joyce GF. Mechanism and utility of an RNA-cleaving DNA enzyme. Biochemistry 1998;37:13330–42.

53. Roy S, Gupta N, Subramanian N, et al. Sequence-specific cleavage of hepatitis C virus RNA by DNAzymes: inhibition of viral RNA translation and replication. J Gen Virol 2008;89:1579–86.
54. Trepanier JB, Tanner JE, Alfieri C. Reduction in intracellular HCV RNA and virus protein expression in human hepatoma cells following treatment with 2′-*O*-methyl-modified anti-core deoxyribozyme. Virology 2008;377:339–44.
55. Trepanier J, Tanner JE, Momparler RL, et al. Cleavage of intracellular hepatitis C RNA in the virus core protein coding region by deoxyribozymes. J Viral Hepat 2006;13:131–8.
56. Altman S, Baer MF, Bartkiewicz M, et al. Catalysis by the RNA subunit of RNase P – a minireview. Gene 1989;82:63–4.
57. Fire A, Xu S, Montgomery MK, et al. Potent and specific genetic interference by double-stranded RNA in *Caenorhabditis elegans*. Nature 1998;391:806–11.
58. Randall G, Rice CM. Interfering with hepatitis C virus RNA replication. Virus Res 2004;102:19–25.
59. Bernstein E, Caudy AA, Hammond SM, et al. Role for a bidentate ribonuclease in the initiation step of RNA interference. Nature 2001;409:363–6.
60. Hammond SM, Bernstein E, Beach D, et al. An RNA-directed nuclease mediates post-transcriptional gene silencing in *Drosophila* cells. Nature 2000;404:293–6.
61. Valencia-Sanchez MA, Liu J, Hannon GJ, et al. Control of translation and mRNA degradation by miRNAs and siRNAs. Genes Dev 2006;20:515–24.
62. Elbashir SM, Harborth J, Lendeckel W, et al. Duplexes of 21-nucleotide RNAs mediate RNA interference in cultured mammalian cells. Nature 2001;411:494–8.
63. Randall G, Grakoui A, Rice CM. Clearance of replicating hepatitis C virus replicon RNAs in cell culture by small interfering RNAs. Proc Natl Acad Sci U S A 2003;100:235–40.
64. Wilson JA, Jayasena S, Khvorova A, et al. RNA interference blocks gene expression and RNA synthesis from hepatitis C replicons propagated in human liver cells. Proc Natl Acad Sci U S A 2003;100:2783–8.
65. Seo MY, Abrignani S, Houghton M, et al. Small interfering RNA-mediated inhibition of hepatitis C virus replication in the human hepatoma cell line Huh-7. J Virol 2003;77:810–2.
66. Takigawa Y, Nagano-Fujii M, Deng L, et al. Suppression of hepatitis C virus replicon by RNA interference directed against the NS3 and NS5B regions of the viral genome. Microbiol Immunol 2004;48:591–8.
67. Prabhu R, Vittal P, Yin Q, et al. Small interfering RNA effectively inhibits protein expression and negative strand RNA synthesis from a full-length hepatitis C virus clone. J Med Virol 2005;76:511–9.
68. Sen A, Steele R, Ghosh AK, et al. Inhibition of hepatitis C virus protein expression by RNA interference. Virus Res 2003;96:27–35.
69. Kanda T, Steele R, Ray R, et al. Small interfering RNA targeted to hepatitis C virus 5′ nontranslated region exerts potent antiviral effect. J Virol 2007;81:669–76.
70. Watanabe T, Umehara T, Yasui F, et al. Liver target delivery of small interfering RNA to the HCV gene by lactosylated cationic liposome. J Hepatol 2007;47:744–50.
71. Kim M, Shin D, Kim SI, et al. Inhibition of hepatitis C virus gene expression by small interfering RNAs using a tri-cistronic full-length viral replicon and a transient mouse model. Virus Res 2006;122:1–10.
72. McCaffrey AP, Meuse L, Pham TT, et al. RNA interference in adult mice. Nature 2002;418:38–9.

73. Jackson AL, Linsley PS. Noise amidst the silence: off-target effects of siRNAs? Trends Genet 2004;20:521–4.
74. Kim VN. MicroRNA biogenesis: coordinated cropping and dicing. Nat Rev Mol Cell Biol 2005;6:376–85.
75. Bentwich I, Avniel A, Karov Y, et al. Identification of hundreds of conserved and nonconserved human microRNAs. Nat Genet 2005;37:766–70.
76. Gottwein E, Cullen BR. Viral and cellular microRNAs as determinants of viral pathogenesis and immunity. Cell Host Microbe 2008;3:375–87.
77. Pedersen IM, Cheng G, Wieland S, et al. Interferon modulation of cellular microRNAs as an antiviral mechanism. Nature 2007;449:919–22.
78. Huang J, Wang F, Argyris E, et al. Cellular microRNAs contribute to HIV-1 latency in resting primary CD4+ T lymphocytes. Nat Med 2007;13:1241–7.
79. Triboulet R, Mari B, Lin YL, et al. Suppression of microRNA-silencing pathway by HIV-1 during virus replication. Science 2007;315:1579–82.
80. Taganov KD, Boldin MP, Baltimore D. MicroRNAs and immunity: tiny players in a big field. Immunity 2007;26:133–7.
81. Chang J, Nicolas E, Marks D, et al. miR-122, a mammalian liver-specific microRNA, is processed from hcr mRNA and may downregulate the high affinity cationic amino acid transporter CAT-1. RNA Biol 2004;1:106–13.
82. Lagos-Quintana M, Rauhut R, Yalcin A, et al. Identification of tissue-specific microRNAs from mouse. Curr Biol 2002;12:735–9.
83. Jopling CL, Yi M, Lancaster AM, et al. Modulation of hepatitis C virus RNA abundance by a liver-specific MicroRNA. Science 2005;309:1577–81.
84. Henke JI, Goergen D, Zheng J, et al. microRNA-122 stimulates translation of hepatitis C virus RNA. EMBO J 2008;27:3300–10.
85. Chang J, Guo JT, Jiang D, et al. Liver-specific microRNA miR-122 enhances the replication of hepatitis C virus in nonhepatic cells. J Virol 2008;82:8215–23.
86. Kutay H, Bai S, Datta J, et al. Downregulation of miR-122 in the rodent and human hepatocellular carcinomas. J Cell Biochem 2006;99:671–8.
87. Mayer G, Jenne A. Aptamers in research and drug development. BioDrugs 2004;18:351–9.
88. Ellington AD, Szostak JW. Selection in vitro of single-stranded DNA molecules that fold into specific ligand-binding structures. Nature 1992;355:850–2.
89. Nishikawa F, Kakiuchi N, Funaji K, et al. Inhibition of HCV NS3 protease by RNA aptamers in cells. Nucleic Acids Res 2003;31:1935–43.
90. Bellecave P, Cazenave C, Rumi J, et al. Inhibition of hepatitis C virus (HCV) RNA polymerase by DNA aptamers: mechanism of inhibition of in vitro RNA synthesis and effect on HCV-infected cells. Antimicrobial Agents Chemother 2008;52: 2097–110.
91. Trahtenherts A, Gal-Tanamy M, Zemel R, et al. Inhibition of hepatitis C virus RNA replicons by peptide aptamers. Antiviral Res 2008;77:195–205.
92. Kakiuchi N, Fukuda K, Nishikawa F, et al. Inhibition of hepatitis C virus serine protease in living cells by RNA aptamers detected using fluorescent protein substrates. Comb Chem High Throughput Screen 2003;6:155–60.
93. Bellecave P, Andreola ML, Ventura M, et al. Selection of DNA aptamers that bind the RNA-dependent RNA polymerase of hepatitis C virus and inhibit viral RNA synthesis in vitro. Oligonucleotides 2003;13:455–63.
94. Kikuchi K, Umehara T, Fukuda K, et al. A hepatitis C virus (HCV) internal ribosome entry site (IRES) domain III-IV-targeted aptamer inhibits translation by binding to an apical loop of domain IIId. Nucleic Acids Res 2005;33: 683–92.

95. Romero-Lopez C, Barroso-delJesus A, Puerta-Fernandez E, et al. Interfering with hepatitis C virus IRES activity using RNA molecules identified by a novel in vitro selection method. Biol Chem 2005;386:183–90.
96. Toulme JJ, Darfeuille F, Kolb G, et al. Modulating viral gene expression by aptamers to RNA structures. Biol Cell 2003;95:229–38.
97. Vo NV, Oh JW, Lai MM. Identification of RNA ligands that bind hepatitis C virus polymerase selectively and inhibit its RNA synthesis from the natural viral RNA templates. Virology 2003;307:301–16.
98. Zimmermann TS, Lee AC, Akinc A, et al. RNAi-mediated gene silencing in non-human primates. Nature 2006;441:111–4.
99. Akhtar S, Benter IF. Nonviral delivery of synthetic siRNAs in vivo. J Clin Invest 2007;117:3623–32.
100. Jackson AL, Bartz SR, Schelter J, et al. Expression profiling reveals off-target gene regulation by RNAi. Nat Biotechnol 2003;21:635–7.
101. Birmingham A, Anderson EM, Reynolds A, et al. 3′ UTR seed matches, but not overall identity, are associated with RNAi off-targets. Nat Methods 2006;3: 199–204.
102. Fedorov Y, Anderson EM, Birmingham A, et al. Off-target effects by siRNA can induce toxic phenotype. RNA 2006;12:1188–96.
103. Jackson AL, Burchard J, Schelter J, et al. Widespread siRNA "off-target" transcript silencing mediated by seed region sequence complementarity. RNA 2006;12:1179–87.
104. Grimm D, Streetz KL, Jopling CL, et al. Fatality in mice due to oversaturation of cellular microRNA/short hairpin RNA pathways. Nature 2006;441:537–41.
105. Sledz CA, Holko M, de Veer MJ, et al. Activation of the interferon system by short-interfering RNAs. Nat Cell Biol 2003;5:834–9.
106. Bridge AJ, Pebernard S, Ducraux A, et al. Induction of an interferon response by RNAi vectors in mammalian cells. Nat Genet 2003;34:263–4.
107. Hornung V, Guenthner-Biller M, Bourquin C, et al. Sequence-specific potent induction of IFN-alpha by short interfering RNA in plasmacytoid dendritic cells through TLR7. Nat Med 2005;11:263–70.
108. Wilson JA, Richardson CD. Hepatitis C virus replicons escape RNA interference induced by a short interfering RNA directed against the NS5b coding region. J Virol 2005;79:7050–8.
109. Konishi M, Wu CH, Kaito M, et al. siRNA-resistance in treated HCV replicon cells is correlated with the development of specific HCV mutations. J Viral Hepat 2006;13:756–61.
110. Henry SD, van der Wegen P, Metselaar HJ, et al. Simultaneous targeting of HCV replication and viral binding with a single lentiviral vector containing multiple RNA interference expression cassettes. Mol Ther 2006;14:485–93.
111. Li H, Li WX, Ding SW. Induction and suppression of RNA silencing by an animal virus. Science 2002;296:1319–21.
112. Li WX, Li H, Lu R, et al. Interferon antagonist proteins of influenza and vaccinia viruses are suppressors of RNA silencing. Proc Natl Acad Sci U S A 2004;101: 1350–5.
113. Lu S, Cullen BR. Adenovirus VA1 noncoding RNA can inhibit small interfering RNA and MicroRNA biogenesis. J Virol 2004;78:12868–76.

Hepatitis C Virus Infection and Immunomodulatory Therapies

Kimberly A. Forde, MD, MHS[a,b], K. Rajender Reddy, MD[a,*]

KEYWORDS

• Hepatitis C infection • Therapy • Immune modulators

Given its global prevalence and the morbidity and mortality of chronic disease associated with it, hepatitis C virus (HCV) infection remains a large-scale and significant health concern. Worldwide, it is estimated that more than 170 million individuals are infected with HCV, with significant variability noted based on geography and route of transmission.[1,2] For example, in the United States, 1.6% of the noninstitutionalized civilian population is estimated to have hepatitis C antibody, representing approximately 3.9 million individuals. Cohorts in other geographic distributions, such as Africa and the United Kingdom, have an estimated population prevalence ranging from 5% to less than1%, respectively.[1,3–5] Once infected, 75% to 85% of those exposed have persistent viremia after 6 months, thus defining a chronically infected state.[6] Chronic infection may progress to cirrhosis, end-stage liver disease, and/or hepatocellular carcinoma. The development of cirrhosis, although variable in population-based cohorts, occurs in approximately 15% to 20% of individuals with chronic infection.[7] Once present, cirrhosis and the manifestations of decompensated disease and hepatocellular carcinoma, occurring at a rate of 1% to 4% per year, result in an increase in morbidity and mortality.[8]

STANDARD OF CARE

The combination of subcutaneously administered pegylated interferon (PEG-IFN) and oral ribavirin is the FDA-approved regimen for the treatment of chronic HCV infection. Combination therapy may result in a sustained virologic response leading to HCV

[a] Division of Gastroenterology, Department of Medicine, University of Pennsylvania, 3400 Spruce Street, 2 Dulles, Philadelphia, PA 19104, USA
[b] Center for Clinical Epidemiology and Biostatistics, Department of Biostatistics and Epidemiology, School of Medicine, University of Pennsylvania, 8th Floor, Blockley Hall, 423 Guardian Drive, Philadelphia, PA 19104, USA
* Corresponding author.
E-mail address: rajender.reddy@uphs.upenn.edu (K.R. Reddy).

Clin Liver Dis 13 (2009) 391–401
doi:10.1016/j.cld.2009.05.007

eradication, with a reduction in risk for cirrhosis, hepatic decompensation, and hepatocellular carcinoma.[9,10] However, the combination of PEG-IFN and ribavirin does not universally result in cure in all patients who undergo treatment. Randomized controlled trials have demonstrated that the response to treatment for chronic HCV is in part based on the genetic makeup of the virus. A sustained virologic response (SVR), defined as the absence of HCV RNA in the serum 6 months after the cessation of HCV therapy, can be achieved in only 42% to 53% of HCV genotype 1 or 4 patients, whereas 78% to 82% of patients infected with HCV genotypes 2 or 3 are cured.[11,12] Demographic factors, including race, ethnicity, body mass index, insulin resistance, and diabetes mellitus, also influence the response to therapy, all resulting in an attenuated response.[13–16] Despite strategies such as high-dose induction therapy and the use of the insulin sensitizers such as metformin and pioglitazone before standard therapy, response rates remain unchanged.[17–19]

In addition to the variable effectiveness of standard of care pharmacotherapy, there are other limitations of treatment with PEG-IFN and ribavirin. Combination therapy results in adverse events, including influenza-like symptoms, cytopenias, psychiatric disturbances such as depression, and dermatologic manifestations. Not only do many of these adverse events require dose reduction in up to 40% of patients in some clinical trials, but in as many as 14% of patients untoward symptoms lead to complete discontinuation of the drug regimen.[11,12,20]

The adverse-event profile of these medications coupled with the reduction in effectiveness noted in patients with certain host factors or viral genotypes underscores the need for the development of more effective and better-tolerated therapies. Many of these new therapeutics may be effective as adjuncts to PEG-IFN and ribavirin combination therapy. However, it is anticipated that some may be efficacious without the need for interferon and/or ribavirin. Although most of the work in new therapeutics against hepatitis C has focused on targeted therapies, the armamentarium also includes therapies that modulate the immune system. This article explores immunomodulatory therapies and highlights their potential use in the treatment of chronic hepatitis C infection.

INTERFERONS

Interferons α, β, and γ were initially recognized for their antiviral properties; however, they have important functions *in vivo* in the modulation of the immune response and up-regulation of immune cell production.[21,22] After binding to its receptor on the cell surface, interferons result in an up-regulation of inflammatory cytokines, augmentation of the T lymphocyte pool, and enhancement of macrophage function.[21]

PEG-IFN α-2a and b are the preparations that are now approved for the treatment of chronic HCV infection. Albinterferon is another formulation of interferon, a recombinant polypeptide composed of interferon α genetically fused to albumin, to exploit the long half-life of this protein.[23] In preclinical studies, this agent demonstrated appropriate antiviral characteristics, and the prolonged half-life for which the agent was formulated was further confirmed. In phase 2 studies, albinterferon, at the dose of 900 μg every 2 weeks, combined with ribavirin was found to be just as efficacious as PEG-IFN and ribavirin, resulting in comparable rates of SVR and adverse events in subjects with genotype 1 chronic HCV infection.[24] Although alternate dosing regimens have been explored, including dosing at four week intervals, 900-μg dosing on a twice-per-month basis not only resulted in a similar antiviral effect as PEG-IFN α-2a but also in improved health-related quality of life throughout the duration of the study. Although higher dosing produced a more desirable early antiviral effect, 1200-μg dosing was associated with no improvement in SVR when compared with other regimens, and resulted in more adverse events and medication discontinuations. Albinterferon α-2b/ribavirin is at present in phase 3 clinical trials to assess noninferiority over PEG-IFN α-2a/ribavirin.[25] Interim results for the primary end points set for genotype 1 and genotype 2/3 subjects suggest that albinterferon has comparable efficacy to PEG-IFN. Further data are awaited regarding the results of these studies.

Long-acting interferon preparations are now being evaluated in clinical trials. One such preparation, locteron (BLX-883), is a controlled-release formulation of unpegylated recombinant interferon α-2b. In a phase 1 clinical trial, locteron was found to produce elevated serum interferon levels for approximately14 days, suggesting the potential for twice-per-month dosing of this drug.[26] Further, this agent had a favorable pharmacokinetic and side-effect profile. In a phase 2a study in HCV genotype 1–treatment naïve subjects, locteron was associated with a significant reduction in HCV viral load and more favorable safety and tolerability.[27] Other interferon preparations, such as (1) PEG-IFN lambda, a novel type III interferon; (2) belerofon, a subcutaneous or oral interferon with an extended half life; (3) omega interferon, a homolog of interferon α and β, which can be administered subcutaneously or by continuous infusion; and (4) maxy-α interferon, a preparation with better immunomodulatory effects, are also in various phases of early clinical trials (**Table 1**).[28–30]

RIBAVIRIN ANALOGS

Recognizing the limitations of interferon monotherapy, ribavirin was added to interferon, given its antiviral properties against several viral pathogens. Although ribavirin was initially recognized only for its antiviral effects, it is now appreciated that ribavirin has immunomodulatory functions as well. Building on the work of many other groups,

Table 1
Immunomodulatory therapies in HCV and current phases of clinical development

Drug Class	Drug	Phase of Development
Interferons	Albinterferon	Phase 3
	Belerofon	Phase 1
	Locteron	Phase 2
	Maxy-alfa	Phase 1
	Omega	Phase 2
	Pegylated interferon λ	Phase 1
Ribavirin analogs	Viramidine (taribavirin)	Phase 3
Antibodies	Bavituximab (monoclonal)	Phase 1
	HCV-AB 68/65 (monoclonal)	Phase 2
	HCV immunoglobulin (polyclonal)	Phase 2
Therapeutic vaccine	ChronVac-C (DNA)	Phase 1/2
	CIGB-230	Phase 1
	GI 5005	Phase 2
	HCV/MF59	Phase 1
	IC41	Phase 2
	PeviPROTM	Phase 1
	TG4040	Phase 1
Toll-like receptors ligand	ANA245 (Isatoribine)	Halted
	CPG 10101 (Actilon)	Halted
	IMO-2125	Phase 1
Thiazolides	Nitazoxanide	Phase 3

Tam and colleagues[31] demonstrated that ribavirin has the ability to polarize the T-cell response *in vivo* toward a T1 profile. Specifically, they demonstrated that, in isolated human T cells, ribavirin exposure resulted in an up-regulation of T1 cytokines, including interleukin-2, interferon γ, and tumor necrosis factor-α, and a down-regulation of T2 cytokines. This finding was illustrated not only at the level of protein expression, but also at the level of mRNA. These findings have changed the view of the anti-HCV effects of ribavirin and helped to explain the potentiation of interferon-based therapy in patients with chronic HCV infection.

In spite of the inherent favorable antiviral and immunomodulatory properties of ribavirin, there is additive toxicity of this agent when coupled with PEG-IFN. As such, investigators have hypothesized that the prodrug of this compound, viramidine, may be associated with fewer adverse events, the most concerning of which is anemia. With standard ribavirin dosing, drug metabolites can be transported into erythrocytes, and subsequently accumulate within these cells. This accumulation is the event that results in hemolytic anemia, an adverse event frequently observed with therapy. In contrast, *in vitro* studies of viramidine have demonstrated that there is less binding of the drug to red blood cells, thereby lending credence to the theory of decreased affinity of this medication for causing anemia. In such studies, viramidine was found to have increased uptake in the liver, with a 32% increase over that seen with conventional oral ribavirin preparations, suggesting the potential for improved efficacy with such specific hepatic targeting.[32]

In an effort to explore the pharmacokinetics of viramidine *in vivo*, Arora and colleagues[33] administered viramidine in escalating doses to subjects with compensated chronic HCV infection. Assessment after 28 days of therapy on 400-mg, 600-mg, or 800-mg dosing showed that all subjects had tolerated therapy with few side effects. The most frequently reported adverse event was that of headaches. In this study, it was also observed that viramidine dosing resulted in lower plasma and red blood cell levels of ribavirin, and as a result, smaller reductions in hemoglobin were noted in the HCV-positive subjects in whom the drug was tested.

As a result of the safety and improved adverse-event profile of viramidine, the efficacy of this prodrug was explored in combination with PEG-IFN in chronically infected HCV subjects. In a phase 2 study, viramidine in combination PEG-IFN was found to yield a similar SVR to standard therapy but with a reduction in the occurrence of anemia.[34] In 2 follow-up phase 3 studies to further evaluate efficacy and safety endpoints, viramidine failed to meet noninferiority endpoints, although again its adverse-event profile was much more favorable than that of weight-based ribavirin. Although efficacy was not substantiated, post hoc analyses suggested an improved response with dosing that approximated 15 to 18 mg/kg body weight.[35] Further studies examining weight-based dosing of viramidine have therefore been suggested.

MONOCLONAL ANTIBODIES

Bavituximab

Bavituximab is a chimeric monoclonal antibody that binds to the phosphotidylserine component of the host cell membrane. After binding has occurred, the immune system is up-regulated and infected host cells targeted. Given that the action of the antibody is against host cell–specific proteins, it is hypothesized that this agent is unlikely to be susceptible to viral resistance.

After successful murine trials with cytomegalovirus and Pichinde virus, a model for Lassa fever, bavituximab was studied in a phase 1 safety and tolerability study.[36] Six patients with chronic HCV infection, who had previously failed combination therapy or relapsed thereafter, were administered an infusion of bavituximab and followed prospectively for a period of 12 weeks. Doses of study drug ranged from 0.1 to 6 mg/kg. Although some adverse events, such as injection site reactions, nausea, and headache, were noted in the study, the drug, on the whole, was deemed safe and was well tolerated by all study participants. A bimodal decrease in HCV RNA was observed in the study participants. The first reduction in viral load was noted 24 hours after infusion and the second on approximately day 4, coinciding with an up-regulation of immune responses specific against HCV. Given early promise noted in this phase I study, clinical trials are still ongoing. Bavituximab is now being studied in subjects with HIV/HCV coinfection.

HCV-AB68

A human monoclonal antibody, HCV-AB68 was generated against E2, an envelope protein of HCV, and was chosen for further exploration because of its activity *in vivo* and ability to neutralize different viral genotypes. This early preclinical success was a segue into a phase 1 clinical study in subjects with chronic HCV infection.[37] In the first phase of this study, a dose-escalation study that explored doses of 0.25 to 40 mg of the study drug in 15 subjects, single infusions of HCV-AB68 were associated with no serious adverse events. Adverse events that were noted in the study were all mild and included headache, fatigue, and myalgias. With respect to antiviral activity, a transient decline in HCV RNA was noted in only 40% of study subjects, with a 2 to 100 fold decrease noted in the first 24 hours after the initial infusion. Such a decrease was not dose dependent and uncorrelated with the baseline viral titer within the respective subject. During the study period, E2 antibody levels did increase after infusions in the highest-dose groups but failed to increase in the lower-dosing groups.

After completion of the phase 1a study, a phase 1b study was conducted to assess the safety, tolerability, and early efficacy of multiple and ascending doses of HCV-AB68.[37] In this study, which enrolled 5 subjects in each of 5 dosing groups (10–120 mg), the drug appeared to be well tolerated in all subjects. There were few adverse events that were of mild to moderate severity and included headache, myalgias, dyspnea, and hypertension. With respect to the antiviral properties of the infusions, increases in anti-E2 antibodies paralleled HCV RNA decreases, with the most noticeable changes noted in the 120-mg-dose group. However, these findings were transient, and a clear dose-response relationship was not demonstrated.

In a phase 2 study, 24 subjects undergoing liver transplantation for HCV-induced cirrhosis were administered HCV-AB68 in escalating doses.[38] In this study, in which subjects received doses ranging from 20 to 240 mg per infusion or placebo, increases in anti-E2 corresponded with decreases in HCV RNA in the 120- and 240-mg-dose groups until about 7 days, when the dosing schedule was lengthened per study protocol. Administration of placebo resulted in more adverse events than active treatment (60% vs 42%, respectively).

To address the concern of mutation in the setting of selective pressure with antibodies directed against 1 viral epitope, researchers have focused on a combination of monoclonal antibodies as well. Eren and collegues[39] combined HCV-AB68 and HCV-AB65, agents which recognize different regions on the HCV E2 protein. They were not only able to demonstrate precipitation of HCV particles and phagocytosis of such particles after complement fixation but also the ability of the antibody combination to inhibit HCV replication and reduce HCV viral load in an HCV-Trimera mouse model. These data are encouraging and may result in further studies of this form of combination therapy in those chronically infected with HCV who are undergoing standard HCV therapy or liver transplantation.

POLYCLONAL ANTIBODIES

Civacir

After the discovery of neutralizing antibodies in immune globulins derived from HCV–positive plasma in chimpanzees and the prevention of infection with its use,[40] hepatitis C immune globulin (HCIG) was evaluated in a cohort of liver transplant recipients. Although an initial pilot study failed to demonstrate the ability of HCIG to prevent recurrence of HCV posttransplant,[41] this immune globulin preparation was retested in this cohort of subjects at higher doses. Three drug groups were explored within a randomized open-label study to evaluate safety endpoints for HCIG.[42] In the study, subjects at 4 centers were randomized to 75 mg/kg of HCIG, 200 mg/kg of HCIG, or no treatment. Before, during, and after a total of 17 infusions at predetermined time points, blood tests, viral kinetics, and liver biopsies were performed in all subjects. Of the 6 subjects enrolled in each treatment arm, almost all had some type of transfusion reaction. The most common symptoms noted were within the trial myalgias, nausea, vomiting, and headache. Six serious adverse events occurred in 3 subjects and included severe transfusion reaction, coagulopathy associated with hypotension, and dehydration associated with gastrointestinal symptomatology.

In spite of the aggressive HCIG transfusion schedule, all HCV antibodies tested, including total, core, and E2, fell in the posttransplantation period. However, the treatment groups maintained higher levels of antibodies in comparison to the control group. With respect to biochemical markers, alanine aminotransferase levels remained lower on average in the treatment groups. Finally, for HCV RNA, there was no inhibition noted in the infusion groups compared with the control group. Additionally, there was no advantage of antibody infusion as seen in the proportion and severity of inflammation noted on liver biopsy. The reason for lack of response in this study was unclear, although the investigators attribute HCIG's failure either to a limitation of dosing or to the ineffective nature of the neutralizing ability of the preparation to control the HCV infection.

VACCINATION

ChronVac-C

ChronVac-C is a naked DNA presently being tested for the treatment of HCV in chronically infected subjects. In a proof-of-concept study, 0.5 mL of ChronVac-C DNA was injected into 12 subjects in varying doses from 167 μg to 1500 μg as 4 monthly doses.[43] After its administration, ChronVac-C was followed by an electrical pulse, a process referred to as electroporation, to allow for passage of the DNA across the host cell membrane. In this study, none of the groups had any report of adverse events. With respect to early efficacy endpoints, however, the 2 highest-dose groups demonstrated a reduction in HCV RNA of greater than $0.5\log_{10}$ for 2 to 10 weeks. Additionally, 3 of the 6 subjects in the 2 highest-dosing groups also had T-cell responses noted at the time of the decline in their HCV viral titers. These data are promising, and phase 1/2a studies are now ongoing.

GI-5005

GI-5005 is a heat-inactivated *Saccharomyces cerevisiae*–based vector that expresses the HCV NS3 and core proteins required for HCV viral replication within the host hepatocyte. GI-5005 targets the immune response in an effort to augment the inflammatory response and promote clearance of HCV-infected cells. In a phase 1b study of 66 chronically HCV-infected subjects who were treatment naïve, partial treatment responders, or treatment relapsers, GI-5005 was administered in 5 weekly doses, followed by 2 monthly injections at various escalating doses.[44] Enrolled study subjects were then followed for 9 months after treatment. Thirty three percent of treated subjects demonstrated an immune response in comparison to none in the placebo group. Further, GI-5005 demonstrated a significant improvement in alanine aminotransferase levels in those treated (29% vs 17% in placebo). Additionally, 13% of the treatment group had a viral titer nadir of $-0.75\log_{10}$ to $-1\log_{10}$. Such reductions were also greatest in the highest-dose group, 20YU (1 YU = 10,000,000 yeast cells). Based on these data, phase 2 clinical trials of this agent are now underway.

Other

Other vaccination-based strategies are on the horizon. IC41 is a T-cell peptide with an added molecular group that primes the immune system for HCV-specific responses. Early favorable results with this agent have spurred early-phase clinical trials. PEV2A/2B are antigens that stimulate CD4 and CD8 cells. A phase 1 clinical trial is now ongoing to assess the safety of these agents in humans. Lastly, dendritic cells primed by HCV core and NS5 proteins may also elicit immune responses in chronic HCV infection. It has been observed in a mouse model that protein-transduced dendritic cells elicit greater T-cell activity than nontransduced cells.[45] It is anticipated that vaccination with these dendritic cells, once tested in humans for safety and tolerability, may become part of the HCV treatment armamentarium.

TOLL-LIKE RECEPTOR LIGANDS

Toll-like receptors (TLRs) are widely dispersed on immune cells and are potent regulators of the innate immune responses. These receptors recognize pathogen-associated patterns and in turn up-regulate the immune response with the production of 1 or more of the following regulatory signals: nuclear factor kB (NF-kB), activator protein-1, and interferon regulatory factors. In chronic hepatitis C infection, the TLR signals are disrupted by viral products in each of the described regulatory pathways.[46] The down-regulation of TLRs observed in chronic HCV infection has lead to the investigation of TLR ligands for the treatment of this viral pathogen.

One such TRL ligand is CPG 10101, also known as Actilon, a TLR9 agonist with documented HCV antiviral properties. Explored first in a phase 1 trial including only healthy adults, CPG 10101 was found to be well tolerated and safe. In a follow-up phase 1b study, such safety and tolerability endpoints were explored in HCV-positive subjects.[47] This study, a multicenter randomized trial, assigned subjects to escalating doses of CPG 10101or placebo given for 4 weeks or given once weekly for 4 weeks. In the 60 subjects treated, a dose-dependent increase was noted in cytokine production, with an increase observed in interferon-γ–inducible protein-19, interferon-α, and 2'5'-oligoadenylate synthetase. Appropriately, decreases in HCV RNA shadowed the up-regulation measured in inflammatory mediators, with the most sizable reduction noted in the highest-dosing group. In the study, 22 of 40 subjects receiving greater than 1 mg of GCP 10101 had a greater than $1\log_{10}$ reduction in their viral titers. Lastly, this agent was again demonstrated to be safe and well tolerated, with minor adverse events, such as flu-like illness and injection-site reactions, being reported throughout the study. Although further studies were conducted, examining the efficacy of this agent in combination with PEG-IFN and ribavirin, further drug development was halted secondary to a lack of efficacy noted in such trials.

Another such TLR agonist is ANA245 or Isatoribine, a TLR7 selective ligand. In a proof-of-concept study,[48] this agent demonstrated a significant decrease in HCV RNA viral load at 800 mg dosing for 7 days. This reduction in HCV RNA was paralleled by an up-regulation of inflammatory cytokines. Further, with ANA245 or Isatoribine, HCV antiviral activity was not only noted with genotype 1 disease but also with others. This agent was also tolerated with few adverse events, all of which were mild to moderate in severity. Future phase clinical trials are awaited to provide additional support for the use of TLR agonists in chronic HCV infection.

THIAZOLIDES

Nitazonide (NTZ), a previously marketed thiazolide used clinically for the treatment of diarrhea resulting from protozoal infections, was noted to have anti-HCV properties in replicon cells.[49] Although the mechanism of action of this therapy is not completely understood, it is thought that NTZ results in an up-regulation of immune function, potentially by exploiting interferon intracellularly. Given the promise in *in vitro* HCV models, NTZ was tested in a safety and efficacy trial in 50 patients. With monotherapy, 7 of 23 subjects treated with NTZ were noted to have an undetectable viral load after 24 weeks of therapy. Although this represents a modest response, the medication was found to be safe at the administered doses for this clinical indication.[50] In larger efficacy trials with the addition of PEG-IFN, NTZ was effective at increasing rapid virologic response, early virologic response, and SVR over standard HCV therapy. A later evaluation of the length of lead-in therapy required for NTZ therapy was conducted, and it was noted that the lead-in could be decreased from the 12 weeks used in previous studies to 4 weeks.[51]

SUMMARY

Combination therapy with PEG-IFN and ribavirin is effective in about 50% of all patients, with even lower rates of SVR noted in certain patient populations. Novel therapies for chronic HCV infection are required to more effectively treat and potentially eradicate this infection. New classes of antiviral medications, specifically those with the ability to modulate the host immune response, demonstrate significant promise and may be considered in the near future in combination with the current standard regimen. As the understanding of the HCV genome increases and the way the virus exploits the host immune response becomes elucidated, drug development will continue to be targeted to providing more tolerable and efficacious therapies.

REFERENCES

1. World Health Organization (WHO). Hepatitis C. Available at: http://www.who.int/mediacentre/factsheets/fs164/en/index.html. Accessed March 1, 2009.
2. Alter MJ, Kruszon-Moran D, Nainan OV, et al. The prevalence of hepatitis C virus infection in the United States, 1988 through 1994. N Engl J Med 1999;341:556–62.
3. Balogun MA, Ramsay ME, Hesketh LM, et al. The prevalence of hepatitis C in England and Wales. J Infect 2002;45:219–26.
4. Mutimer DJ, Harrison RF, O'Donnell KB, et al. Hepatitis C virus infection in the asymptomatic British blood donor. J Viral Hepat 1995;2:47–53.
5. Booth JC, Brown JL, Thomas HC. The management of chronic hepatitis C virus infection. Gut 1995;37:449–54.
6. Hoofnagle JH. Hepatitis C: the clinical spectrum of disease. Hepatology 1997;26:15S–20S.

7. Liang TJ, Rehermann B, Seeff LB, et al. Pathogenesis, natural history, treatment, and prevention of hepatitis C. Ann Intern Med 2000;132:296–305.
8. El-Serag HB. Hepatocellular carcinoma and hepatitis C in the United States. Hepatology 2002;36:S74–83.
9. Nishiguchi S, Kuroki T, Nakatani S, et al. Randomised trial of effects of interferon-alpha on incidence of hepatocellular carcinoma in chronic active hepatitis C with cirrhosis. Lancet 1995;346:1051–5.
10. Effect of interferon-alpha on progression of cirrhosis to hepatocellular carcinoma: a retrospective cohort study. International Interferon-alpha Hepatocellular Carcinoma Study Group. Lancet 1998;351:1535–9.
11. Fried MW, Shiffman ML, Reddy KR, et al. Peginterferon alfa-2a plus ribavirin for chronic hepatitis C virus infection. N Engl J Med 2002;347:975–82.
12. Manns MP, McHutchison JG, Gordon SC, et al. Peginterferon alfa-2b plus ribavirin compared with interferon alfa-2b plus ribavirin for initial treatment of chronic hepatitis C: a randomised trial. Lancet 2001;358:958–65.
13. Muir AJ, Bornstein JD, Killenberg PG. Peginterferon alfa-2b and ribavirin for the treatment of chronic hepatitis C in blacks and non-Hispanic whites. N Engl J Med 2004;350:2265–71.
14. Rodriguez-Torres M, Jeffers LJ, Sheikh MY, et al. Peginterferon alfa-2a and ribavirin in Latino and non-Latino whites with hepatitis C. N Engl J Med 2009; 360:257–67.
15. Bressler BL, Guindi M, Tomlinson G, et al. High body mass index is an independent risk factor for nonresponse to antiviral treatment in chronic hepatitis C. Hepatology 2003;38:639–44.
16. Romero-Gomez M, Del Mar Viloria M, Andrade RJ, et al. Insulin resistance impairs sustained response rate to peginterferon plus ribavirin in chronic hepatitis C patients. Gastroenterology 2005;128:636–41.
17. Romero-Gomez M, Diago M, Andrade RJ, et al. Metformin with peginterferon alfa-2a and ribavirin in the treatment of naive genotype 1 chronic hepatitis C patients with insulin resistance (TRIC-1): final results of a randomized and double-blinded trial [abstract LB6]. Hepatology 2008;48(Suppl 1):380A.
18. Conjeevaram HS, Burant CF, McKenna B, et al. A randomized, double-blind, placebo-controlled study of PPAR-gamma agonist pioglitazone given in combination with peginterferon and ribavirin in patients with genotype-1 chronic hepatitis C [abstract]. Hepatology 2008;48(Suppl 1):384A.
19. Elgouhari HM, Cesario KB, Lopez R, et al. Pioglitazone improves early virologic kinetic response to Peg IFN/RBV combination therapy in hepatitis C genotype 1 naïve patients [abstract]. Hepatology 2008;48(Suppl 1):383A.
20. Hadziyannis SJ, Sette H Jr, Morgan TR, et al. Peginterferon-alpha2a and ribavirin combination therapy in chronic hepatitis C: a randomized study of treatment duration and ribavirin dose. Ann Intern Med 2004;140:346–55.
21. Tompkins WA. Immunomodulation and therapeutic effects of the oral use of interferon-alpha: mechanism of action. J Interferon Cytokine Res 1999;19:817–28.
22. Brunton LL. Goodman and Gilman's the pharmacologic basis of therapeutics. The McGraw-Hill Companies; USA: 2006.
23. Subramanian GM, Fiscella M, Lamouse-Smith A, et al. Albinterferon alpha-2b: a genetic fusion protein for the treatment of chronic hepatitis C. Nat Biotechnol 2007;25:1411–9.
24. Zeuzem S, Yoshida EM, Benhamou Y, et al. Albinterferon alfa-2b dosed every two or four weeks in interferon-naive patients with genotype 1 chronic hepatitis C. Hepatology 2008;48:407–17.

25. Rustgi VK. Albinterferon alfa-2b, a novel fusion protein of human albumin and human interferon alfa-2b, for chronic hepatitis C. Curr Med Res Opin 2009; 25(4):991–1002.
26. De Leede LG, Humphries JE, Bechet AC, et al. Novel controlled-release Lemna-derived IFN-alpha2b (Locteron): pharmacokinetics, pharmacodynamics, and tolerability in a phase I clinical trial. J Interferon Cytokine Res 2008;28:113–22.
27. Dzyublyk I, Yegorova T, Moroz L, et al. Phase 2a study to evaluate the safety and tolerability and anti-viral of 4 doses of a novel, controlled-release interferon alfa-2b (Locteron) given every 2 weeks for 12 weeks in treatment-naive patients with chronic hepatitis C (genotype 1) [abstract LB10]. Hepatology 2007;46(Suppl 1): 863A.
28. Lawitz E, Zaman A, Muir A, et al. Interim results from a phase 1b dose-escalation study of 4 weeks of peg-interferon lambda (PEG-RIL-29) treatment in subjects with hepatitis C virus (HCV) genotype 1 with prior virologic response and relapse to peginterferon alfa and ribavirin [abstract 170]. Hepatology 2008;48(Suppl 1): 385A.
29. Novozhenov V, Zakharova N, Vinogradova E, et al. J.M. Phase 2 study of omega interferon alone or in combination with ribavirin in subjects with chronic hepatitis C genotype-1 infection [abstract 11]. J Hepatol 2007;46(Suppl 1):S8.
30. Kronenberger B, Welsch C, Forestier N, et al. Novel hepatitis C drugs in current trials. Clin Liver Dis 2008;12:529–55, viii.
31. Tam RC, Pai B, Bard J, et al. Ribavirin polarizes human T cell responses towards a Type 1 cytokine profile. J Hepatol 1999;30:376–82.
32. Lin CC, Yeh LT, Vitarella D, et al. Viramidine, a prodrug of ribavirin, shows better liver-targeting properties and safety profiles than ribavirin in animals. Antivir Chem Chemother 2003;14:145–52.
33. Arora S, Xu C, Teng A, et al. Ascending multiple-dose pharmacokinetics of viramidine, a prodrug of ribavirin, in adult subjects with compensated hepatitis C infection. J Clin Pharmacol 2005;45:275–85.
34. Gish RG, Arora S, Rajender Reddy K, et al. Virological response and safety outcomes in therapy-naive patients treated for chronic hepatitis C with taribavirin or ribavirin in combination with pegylated interferon alfa-2a: a randomized, phase 2 study. J Hepatol 2007;47:51–9.
35. Marcellin P, Lurie Y, Rodrigues-Torres M, et al. The safety and efficacy of taribavirin plus pegylated interferon alfa-2a versus ribavirin plus pegylated interferon alfa-2a in therapy-naive patients infected with HCV: phase 3 results [abstract 10]. J Hepatol 2007;46(Suppl 1):S7.
36. Godofsky E, Shan J. Phase I singe dose study of bavituximab, a chimeric anti-phosphatidylserine monoclonal antibody, in subjects with chronic hepatitis C [abstract 127]. Hepatology 2006;44(Suppl 1):236A.
37. Galun E, Terrault NA, Eren R, et al. Clinical evaluation (Phase I) of a human monoclonal antibody against hepatitis C virus: safety and antiviral activity. J Hepatol 2007;46:37–44.
38. Schiano TD, Charlton M, Younossi Z, et al. Monoclonal antibody HCV-AbXTL68 in patients undergoing liver transplantation for HCV: results of a phase 2 randomized study. Liver Transpl 2006;12:1381–9.
39. Eren R, Landstein D, Terkieltaub D, et al. Preclinical evaluation of two neutralizing human monoclonal antibodies against hepatitis C virus (HCV): a potential treatment to prevent HCV reinfection in liver transplant patients. J Virol 2006;80: 2654–64.

40. Yu MY, Bartosch B, Zhang P, et al. Neutralizing antibodies to hepatitis C virus (HCV) in immune globulins derived from anti-HCV-positive plasma. Proc Natl Acad Sci U S A 2004;101:7705–10.
41. Willems J, Ede M, Marotta P, et al. Anti-HCV human immunogobulins for the prevention of graft infection in HCV-related liver transplantation, a pilot study. J Hepatol 2002;36(Suppl 1):32 [abstract 96].
42. Davis GL, Nelson DR, Terrault N, et al. A randomized, open-label study to evaluate the safety and pharmacokinetics of human hepatitis C immune globulin (Civacir) in liver transplant recipients. Liver Transpl 2005;11:941–9.
43. Sallberg M, Frelin L, Diepolder H, et al. A first clinical trial of therapeutic vaccination using naked DNA delivered by in vivo electroporation shows antiviral effects in patients with chronic hepatitis C [abstract 43]. Journal of Hepatology 2009;50(Suppl 1):S18–9.
44. Schiff E, Everson G, Tsai N, et al. HCV-specific cellular immunity, RNA reductions, and normalization of ALT in chronic HCV subjects after treatment with GI-5005, a yeast-based immunotherapy targeting NS3 and core: a randomized, double-blind, placebo controlled phase 1B study. Hepatology 2007;46(Suppl 1):816A [abstract 1304].
45. Kuzushita N, Gregory SH, Monti NA, et al. Vaccination with protein-transduced dendritic cells elicits a sustained response to hepatitis C viral antigens. Gastroenterology 2006;130:453–64.
46. Seki E, Brenner DA. Toll-like receptors and adaptor molecules in liver disease: update. Hepatology 2008;48:322–35.
47. McHutchison JG, Bacon BR, Gordon SC, et al. Phase 1B, randomized, double-blind, dose-escalation trial of CPG 10101 in patients with chronic hepatitis C virus. Hepatology 2007;46:1341–9.
48. Horsmans Y, Berg T, Desager JP, et al. Isatoribine, an agonist of TLR7, reduces plasma virus concentration in chronic hepatitis C infection. Hepatology 2005;42: 724–31.
49. Korba BE, Montero AB, Farrar K, et al. Nitazoxanide, tizoxanide and other thiazolides are potent inhibitors of hepatitis B virus and hepatitis C virus replication. Antiviral Res 2008;77:56–63.
50. Rossignol JF, Kabil SM, El-Gohary Y, et al. Clinical trial: randomized, double-blind, placebo-controlled study of nitazoxanide monotherapy for the treatment of patients with chronic hepatitis C genotype 4. Aliment Pharmacol Ther 2008; 28:574–80.
51. Rossignol J, Elfert A, Keeffe E. Evaluation of a 4 week lead-in phase with nitazoxanide (NTZ) prior to peginterferon (PEGIFN) plus NTZ for treatment of chronic hepatitis C: final report [abstract 87]. Hepatology 2008;48(Suppl 1):344A.

Cyclophilin Inhibitors

Philippe A. Gallay, PhD

KEYWORDS

- Hepatitis C virus (HCV) • Cyclophilins
- Cyclosporine A derivatives • Inhibitors • Isomerase

The hepatitis C virus (HCV) is the main contributing agent of acute and chronic liver diseases worldwide.[1] Primary infection is often asymptomatic or associated with mild symptoms. However, individuals with a persistent infection develop an increased risk of chronic liver diseases such as cirrhosis and hepatocellular carcinoma.[1] There are approximately 170 million people chronically infected and 3 to 4 million new cases of infection each year.[2,3] In the developed world, HCV is responsible for 50% to 75% of all cases of liver cancer and accounts for two-thirds of all liver transplants.[4]

LIMITATION OF CURRENT THERAPY

The percentage of patients chronically infected with HCV who have reached sustained antiviral response (SVR) has increased since the introduction of pegylated IFN-alpha (pIFNa) and ribavirin (RBV) treatment.[5,6] SVR is defined as an undetectable HCV RNA (polymerase chain reaction [PCR]) for 24 weeks after completion of therapy and is associated with a durable viral clearance in more than 99.8% of cases. However, the current standard pIFNa/RBV therapy not only has a low success rate (about 50%)[7,8] but is often associated with serious side effects including flulike illness, fever, fatigue, hematological disease, anemia, leucopenia, thrombocytopenia, alopecia, and depression.[9] The morbidity and mortality rates associated with HCV are predicted to increase in the coming years, and more efficacious and tolerable therapies are urgently required, particularly for the increasing proportion of patients, who are resistant to pIFNa/RBV treatment.[10,11] The low success rate of the pIFNa/RBV treatment arises from various factors ranging from differences in HCV genotypes and variation within specific patient populations. Among the 6 HCV genotypes, genotype 1 is the most prevalent in Europe and North America and is the most difficult to treat; it represents the greatest unmet treatment need.[12] Certain patient populations are difficult to treat including nonresponders to prior pIFNa/RBV treatment, patients with severe liver fibrosis or cirrhosis, those of African American ethnicity, individuals coinfected with HIV, and patients with high alcohol consumption, fatty liver, or insulin

This is publication no. 19970-IMM from the Department of Immunology and Microbial Science, The Scripps Research Institute, La Jolla, CA.
Department of Immunology and Microbial Science, The Scripps Research Institute, 10550 N. Torrey Pines Road, La Jolla, CA 92037, USA
E-mail address: gallay@scripps.edu

Clin Liver Dis 13 (2009) 403–417
doi:10.1016/j.cld.2009.05.002
liver.theclinics.com
1089-3261/09/$ – see front matter

resistance.[1,13–20] For example, response rates in African American patients with genotype 1 HCV have been shown to be as low as 6% to 26%, and 50% in those with genotypes 2 or 3.[16,17] This is compared with overall cure rates of 45% to 55% for genotype 1 and more than 75% to 80% in genotypes 2 and 3 for non-Hispanic whites.[21–24] Given that there are no approved alternative treatments available for patients who fail to respond to the pIFNa/RBV treatment, there is an urgent need for the development of new anti-HCV agents with novel mechanisms of antiviral action.

ALTERNATIVE APPROACHES: STAT-C DRUGS

One approach to identify new anti-HCV agents is to target specific steps of the HCV life cycle. These agents are termed "specifically targeted antiviral therapy for HCV" or STAT-C drugs.[25,26] Among the most promising new anti-HCV agents in clinical development are the protease and polymerase inhibitors (**Fig. 1**). Another new promising strategy consists of targeting host factors such as cyclophilins (Cyps), which are involved in HCV replication (see **Fig. 1**).

Cyclophilin Inhibitors in Clinical and Preclinical Studies

A new class of oral inhibitors that targets the host factors involved in HCV has arisen from clinical and in vitro studies using the immunosuppressive drug cyclosporine A (CsA). The most likely mechanism for CsA reduction of HCV replication is by neutralization of Cyps.

In vitro studies provided evidence that CsA prevents HCV RNA replication and HCV protein production in an IFNa-independent manner.[27–31] CsA was reported to be clinically effective against HCV.[32] Controlled trials showed that a combination of CsA with IFNa is more effective than IFNa alone, especially in patients with a high viral load.[33,34] However, the immunosuppressive anticalcineurin activity of CsA limits its use in the clinic as an anti-HCV agent. CsA exerts this anti-HCV activity independently of its immunosuppressive activity. In vitro studies have demonstrated that nonimmunosuppressive CsA derivatives also block HCV RNA and protein production.[30,35–38] There are 3 nonimmunosuppressive Cyp inhibitors currently being evaluated in preclinical and clinical studies: Debio 025, NIM811 and SCY-635 (**Figs. 1** and **2**).

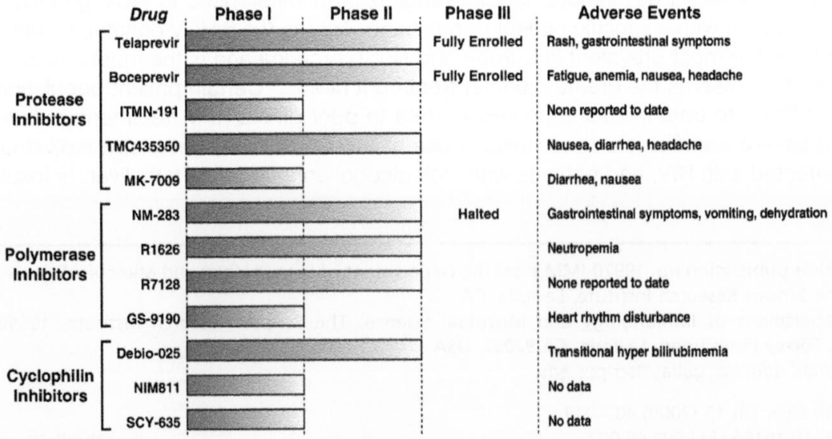

Fig. 1. Cyclophilin, polymerase and protease inhibitors currently in clinical studies.

	Structure	Immunosuppression Activity (IL-2 inhibition)	CypA PPlase Inhibition (Ki)	Anti-HCV Activity (EC_{50})
Cyclosporin A	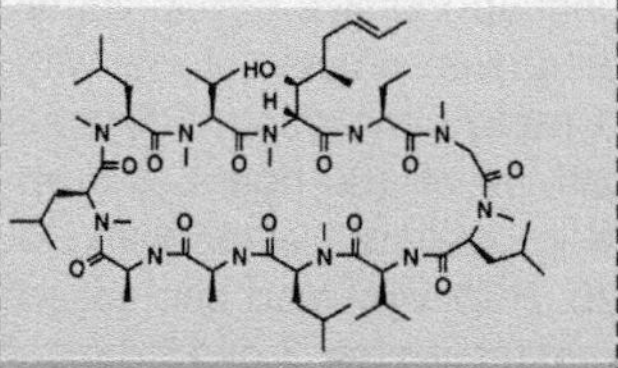	0.006 µg/mL	9.79 nM	0.3 µM
NIM811	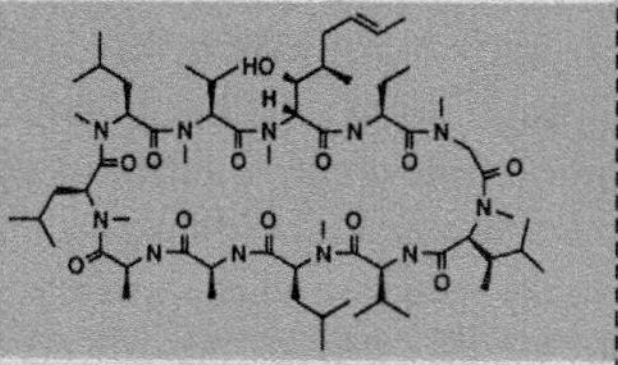	>10 µg/mL	2.11 nM	0.06 µM
Debio-025	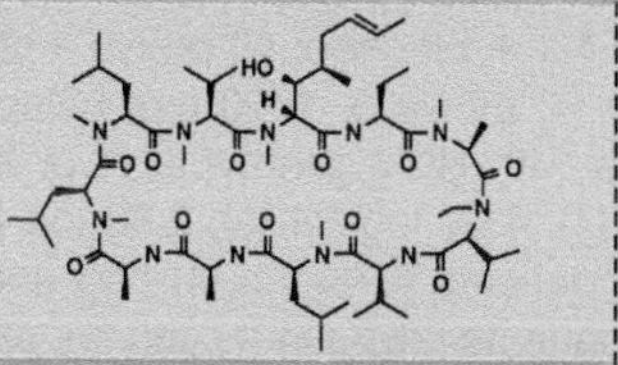	21.5 µg/mL	0.34 nM	0.04 µM
SCY-635	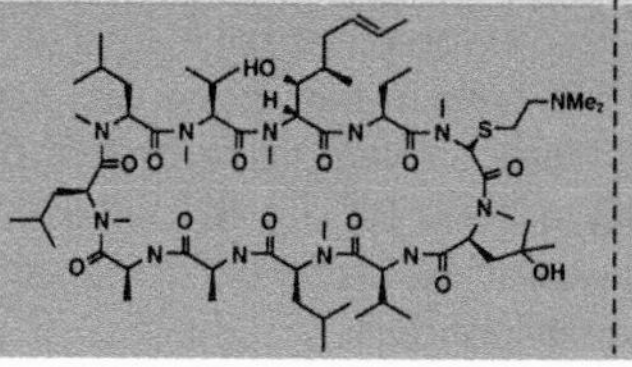	13 µg/mL	1.8 nM	0.1 µM

Fig. 2. Anti-immunosuppressive, anti-PPIase and anti-HCV activity of Cyp inhibitors. An in vitro assay for immunosuppression: IL-2 promoter activation on T cell stimulation was determined in a Jurkat T cell line containing the beta-galactosidase gene as a reporter under IL-2 promoter control.[8] PPIase inhibition assay. The inhibition of the PPIase activity of CypA was used to compare the inhibitory potential of cyclosporines as an indication of their binding affinity to CypA. The PPIase activity was measured in a chymotrypsin-coupled spectrophotometry assay based on the method described previously.[31] Antiviral efficacy of Cyp inhibitors was measured as described previously.[37]

Debio 025

Debio 025, a synthetic Cyp inhibitor derived from CsA, is being tested in humans as a potential anti-HCV drug. Debio 025 binds strongly to Cyps, host cell proteins believed to confer a replication advantage to HCV (see **Fig. 2**). In vitro studies have demonstrated that Debio 025 is active at the submicromolar range in the HCV replicon and shows the unique ability to clear hepatoma cells from their HCV replicon when used alone or in combination with other antivirals.[37] The combination of Debio 025 with IFNa, RBV, and STAT-C drugs, such as the protease inhibitor VX-950, the nucleoside polymerase inhibitor 2′-CMeCyt and the non-nucleoside polymerase inhibitor JT-16, results in additive to slightly synergistic antiviral effects.[34] Resistant replicon cells, selected by cell passage in the presence of increasing concentrations of Debio 025, remain sensitive to protease or polymerase inhibitors and IFNa.[34] Conversely, Debio 025 remains fully active against wild-type HCV and HCV replicons resistant to protease or polymerase inhibitors.[34] The emergence of resistant variants to protease inhibitors (VX-950 and BILN2061) or polymerase inhibitors (JT-16 and

R1479) is restrained by Debio 025.[34] Debio 025 in combination with pIFNa is also potent against HCV in a chimeric mouse model.[38]

Debio 025 was the first oral nonimmunosuppressive Cyp inhibitor to enter clinical trials. A 15-day double-blind, placebo-controlled phase I study, with twice daily oral doses (1200 mg) of Debio 025 showed rapid absorption, with peak plasma levels reached after 2 hours and a terminal half-life of 100 hours. A drop in the maximal HCV RNA level of 3.6 log was observed in patients treated with Debio 025.[39] In 15 out of 16 subjects treated with Debio 025, HCV viral load decreased by more than 2 log. In 3 patients the virus became undetectable after 8 or 15 days. All 3 HCV genotypes (1, 3 and 4) identified in the study responded well to the dose administered and no patient developed a viral breakthrough during the treatment, suggesting that Debio 025 has a high barrier for resistance. However, transient hyperbilirubinemia led to the discontinuation of treatment in some patients.[39] More recently, the efficacy of Debio 025 in combination with pIFNa in chronic hepatitis C patients was evaluated in a phase II study.[40,41] The study included 90 participants who received 1 of the following treatments for 29 days: (1) pIFNa + placebo; (2) pIFNa + 200 mg/d Debio 025; (3) pIFNa + 600 mg/d Debio 025; (4) pIFNa + 1000 mg/d Debio 025; and (5) 1000 mg/d Debio 025. Among patients with HCV genotypes 1 or 4, reductions in HCV RNA at day 29 were 4.75 log for (4), 4.61 log for (3), 2.49 log for (1), 2.20 log for (5), and 1.8 log for (2). Eight of 12 patients (67%) in (4) had undetectable viral load at day 29, compared with 3 of 12 patients (25%) in (1) and (5). Among genotype 2 or 3 patients, 4 out of 6 (67%) achieved undetectable HCV RNA with Debio 025 monotherapy. The reduction of HCV RNA levels in this group was 4.22 log. At lower doses, the safety profile of Debio 025 was comparable to that of placebo. Five of 24 patients (21%), who received 1000 mg of Debio 025 developed reversible increases in indirect bilirubin resulting in hyperbilirubinemia. Debio 025 is currently being evaluated in another phase II study in IFN nonresponders.

NIM811

NIM811 was the first synthesized Cyp inhibitor derived from CsA found to be devoid of immunosuppressive activity. NIM811 binds to Cyps with higher affinity than CsA[26] (see **Fig. 2**). Rosenwirth and colleagues[42] were the first to demonstrate a potent antiviral activity of NIM811 against human immunodeficiency virus type 1 (HIV-1). Most recently, NIM811, like Debio 025, was found to exert anti-HCV activities in vitro.[26,28,36] Specifically, Lin and colleagues[28] showed that NIM811 efficiently reduced HCV RNA levels in replicon cells with a 50% inhibitory concentration of 0.66 μM at 48 hours. A drop in viral RNA greater 3 log was achieved after treating cells with 1 μM NIM811 for 9 days. The combination of NIM811 with IFNa significantly enhanced anti-HCV activities without causing any increase in cytotoxicity.[28] The combination of NIM811 with other virus-specific inhibitors was recently investigated in HCV replicon cells. All combinations led to more pronounced antiviral effects than any single agent, with no significant increase in cytotoxicity.[28] The combination of NIM811 with a nucleoside (NM107) or a non-nucleoside (thiophene-2-carboxylic acid) polymerase inhibitor was synergistic, whereas the combination with a protease inhibitor (BILN2061) was additive.[36] These results are in accordance with recent Debio 025 results, which showed that the combination of Debio 025 with either RBV or NS3 protease or NS5B polymerase inhibitors resulted in an additive antiviral activity in short-term antiviral assays.[36] Resistant clones were selected in vitro with NIM811, NM107, or BILN2061. Lin and colleagues[36] found that it was much more difficult to develop resistance against NIM811 than against protease and polymerase inhibitors. This significant delay of resistance development against NIM811 was also observed for CsA and Debio 025.[34] Specifically, Neyts and colleagues[36] showed that for several HCV inhibitors such as BILN2061, HCV-796, thiophene carboxylic acid, and benzothiadiazines, drug-resistant variants were rapidly selected when replicon cells were cultured in the presence of high drug concentrations (25- to 125-fold median effective concentration [EC_{50}]). In sharp contrast, resistance to Debio 025 could only be selected following a lengthy stepwise selection procedure. One can speculate that developing resistances that obviate the need for host Cyps in HCV replication represents a major challenge for the virus. No cross-resistance was observed between NIM811 and NM107 or BILN2061.[36] NIM811 was highly effective at blocking the emergence of resistance when used in combination with the HCV protease or polymerase inhibitors.[36] The NIM811 and Debio 025 data illustrate the advantage of combining inhibitors targeting viral and host proteins. A phase I escalating dose study to assess safety, pharmacokinetic, and pharmacodynamic profiles following NIM811 administration in patients with hepatitis C genotype 1 has started. The study period is 14 days with NIM811/placebo administration together with pIFNa, with the option to continue on pIFN/RBV for up to 48 weeks. No clinical data have yet been reported.

SCY-635

SCY-635, the latest nonimmunosuppressive Cyp inhibitor derived from CsA, was recently evaluated in preclinical studies and was found to exhibit favorable anti-HCV properties (see **Figs. 1** and **2**). SCY-635, like NIM811 and Debio 025, binds to Cyps with a higher affinity than CsA[43] (see **Fig. 2**). Hopkins and colleagues[43] demonstrated that the in vitro antiviral, pharmacokinetic, and cytotoxic profiles of SCY-635 are superior to those of CsA. The antiviral effects of the combination of SCY-635 with IFNa on HCV replicon cells are additive to synergistic.[35] SCY-635 is currently being evaluated in a 15-day phase I randomized, double-blind, placebo-controlled, multidose study in genotype 1 patients (see **Fig. 1**). Preliminary clinical data suggest that SCY-635 was well tolerated and triggered a significant reduction of plasma HCV RNA levels. However, the full results of the study have not yet been presented.

CYCLOSPORINE A AND CYCLOPHILINS

In 1970, Thiele isolated the fungus *Tolypocladium inflatum* from soil samples.[44] Two *Tolypocladium inflatum* metabolites named cyclosporin A (CsA) and C (CsC) were then tested for various pharmacologic activities. Out of all the pharmacologic tests, only 1 generated a positive result. This was a test for immunosuppression.[44] Further experiments showed that CsA specifically blocked the proliferation of lymphocytes, launching a new era in immunopharmacology.[44] It was the first immunosuppressive drug allowing specific immunoregulation of T cells without excessive toxicity. In 1976, Borel discovered that CsA selectively suppresses T cell immunity.[44] This led to further investigations into the properties of CsA involving further immunologic tests, structure and synthesis analyses. In 1983, CsA was approved for clinical use to prevent graft rejection in transplantation.[45]

In 1984, cyclophilin A (CypA) was isolated by Handschumacher and colleagues[46] from bovine thymocytes as a protein that specifically binds CsA. Further studies demonstrated that CypA is the in vivo target for CsA allowing repression of immune-mediated tissue rejection by inhibition of the activation of specific subsets of T lymphocytes.[45] The same year, Fischer and colleagues[47] identified an activity catalyzing the *cis* to *trans* interconversion of the proline-containing peptides (**Fig. 3**). This new type of enzyme was classified as peptidyl-prolyl *cis-trans*-isomerases (PPIases).[48] The peptide bond generally exists in 2 stable isomeric forms: *cis* and *trans*.[49] The ribosome synthesizes peptide bonds in the lower energy state *trans*

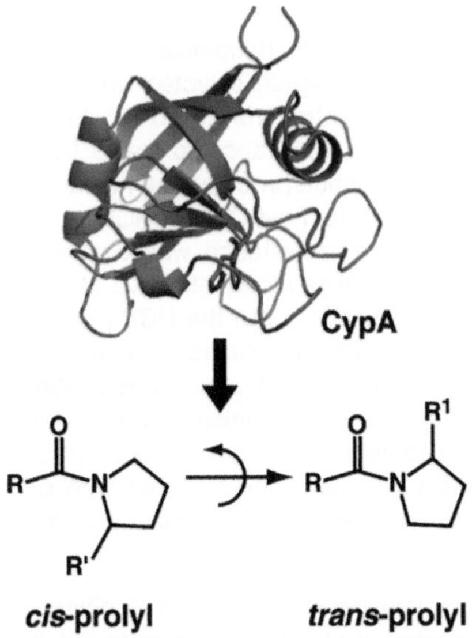

Fig. 3. Peptidyl-prolyl *cis-trans* isomerase action of cyclophilin A. Cyclophilin A is an in vitro catalyst of the peptide bond rotation on the amino side of proline residues.

peptide bond form, which is sterically favored with its side chains 180 degrees opposite each other.[50] However, bonds preceding each proline (peptidyl-prolyl bonds) also occur in the *cis* form in unfolded and native proteins, with the side chains adjacent to each other.[50] Isomerization to the *cis* form is required for de novo protein folding, protein restructuring, and refolding processes following cellular membrane traffic. Spontaneous *cis/trans* isomerization of peptidyl-prolyl bonds is a slow process at room temperature that does not require free energy. Thus, this isomerization represents a rate-limiting step in the refolding of chemically denatured proteins.[51] About 5 years later, Fischer and colleagues[52] discovered that the PPIase activity that they previously identified as an in vitro catalyst of the peptide bond rotation on the amino side of proline residues and folding of proteins, was the CypA protein that Handschumacher isolated in 1984. CsA binding to the hydrophobic pocket of CypA neutralizes the isomerase activity of CypA.[53,54] Bacteria, fungi, insects, plants, and mammals contain Cyps, which all have PPIase activity and are structurally conserved.[55] To date, 16 Cyp members have been identified and 7 major members are found in humans: CypA, CypB, CypC, CypD, CypE, Cyp40, and CypNK.[55] All Cyps contain a common domain of 109 amino acids, called the Cyp-like domain, which is surrounded by domains specific to each Cyp member that dictate their cellular compartmentalization and function.[55] CypA homologs were found to be responsible for CsA toxicity in *Saccharomyces cerevisiae* and *Neurospora crassa*.[55,56] The existence of knockout mice[57] and knockout human cell lines[58] suggest that CypA is optional for cell growth and survival. Although PPIase CypA was identified 25 years ago, its true cellular function remains unknown.

CYCLOPHILINS AND VIRUSES

It is well established that host proteins highly regulate the viral life cycles. Because cellular chaperones and enzymes control the correct folding of host proteins, one could assume that they also control the correct folding of viral proteins. This assumption seems to be true for 2 prime human pathogens: HIV-1[59] and HCV. In 1993, Luban and colleagues,[60] using the yeast 2-hybrid system, identified a direct and specific interaction between CypA and HIV-1 Gag. One year later, 2 independent studies elegantly demonstrated that CypA-Gag interactions are critical for HIV-1 replication in human cells.[61–63] Specifically, Thali and colleagues[61] showed that CsA, by preventing CypA-Gag interactions, inhibits HIV-1 infection. Moreover, Franke and colleagues[62] showed that the introduction of mutations in the CypA-binding region of Gag, which also prevents CypA-Gag interactions, decreases HIV-1 infection of human cells. Further supporting the notion that HIV-1 requires CypA to replicate, several studies showed that CypA-knockout and -knockdown human cells poorly support HIV-1 replication.[59,64,65]

Similar to HIV-1, several lines of evidence indicate that Cyps also play a key role in HCV replication. The first evidence was provided in 2003 by Shimotohno and colleagues,[30] who demonstrated that CsA and nonimmunosuppressive CsA derivates suppress HCV replication in vitro. The CsA-mediated HCV inhibition was rapidly confirmed by Watanabe and colleagues.[29] The first link between CsA-mediated inhibition and Cyps was provided by Shimotohno and colleagues,[65] who presented several lines of evidence that CypB is critical for HCV replication. Specifically, they showed that small interfering RNA interference (siRNA)-mediated reduction of endogenous CypB expression inhibits HCV replication.[65] They also presented data that suggest that CypB, by binding to the NS5B, stimulates the binding of NS5B to the viral RNA.[65] Moreover, they presented data that suggest that preventing NS5B-CypB interactions diminishes HCV replication.[65] Based on these findings, CypB was proposed to act as a stimulatory regulator of NS5B in the HCV replication machinery.[65,66] Supporting the notion that Cyps modulate HCV replication, Watanabe and colleagues[67] showed that knocking down the expression of CypA, CypB and CypC by siRNA suppresses HCV replication. However, more recently, Tang and colleagues[68] showed that silencing CypB or CypC expression by siRNA had no significant effect on HCV replication, whereas silencing CypA profoundly blocked HCV replication. Re-expression of CypA in the CypA-silenced hepatocytes rescued HCV replication, demonstrating the importance of CypA in HCV replication.[68] Thus, although there was a growing body of evidence that Cyps control HCV replication in human hepatocytes, a major disagreement existed on the respective roles of Cyp members in HCV replication. Specifically, Watashi and colleagues[65] demonstrated that CypB, but not CypA, assists HCV replication, whereas Yang and colleagues[68] demonstrated the exact opposite. Moreover, Nakagawa and colleagues[67] demonstrated that CypA, CypB, and CypC are all required for HCV replication. However, 2 independent studies from the Bartenschlager laboratory[69] and from our laboratory[70] recently re-examined the respective contributions of Cyp members to HCV replication using stable Cyp-knockdown cell lines. These 2 studies confirmed Tang's results: CypA represents the main Cyp member that HCV exploits to replicate in hepatocytes.[69,70] Thus, to date, 3 independent studies have demonstrated convincingly that HCV replication relies mainly on host cytosolic CypA. Further work is required to exclude (or not) the possibility that other Cyps, such as CypB, in concert with CypA, also assist HCV replication.

MECHANISMS OF ACTION OF CYCLOPHILIN INHIBITORS

The current hypothesis is that nonimmunosuppressive Cyp inhibitors, by specifically targeting intracellular Cyps, block HCV replication.[68–70] However, several critical questions remain to be answered. First, how do Cyps assist HCV replication? To date, auxiliary and essential biochemical functions can be attributed to Cyps. The auxiliary function is characterized by polypeptide sequestration using extended catalytic subsites of the enzyme, whereas catalysis essentially requires direct participation of active site residues.[71] The authors and others recently demonstrated that when we mutate residues that reside in the hydrophobic pocket of CypA (histidine or arginine in positions 126 and R55, respectively), where the proline-containing peptide substrates bind, the resulting CypA mutants fail to restore HCV replication.[69,70] The simplest hypothesis for the mechanism of action of CypA in the HCV life cycle is that it catalyzes a *trans* to *cis* or a *cis* to *trans* isomerization of a peptidyl-prolyl bond in a viral or host protein critical for HCV replication. The observation that Cyp inhibitors (Debio 025, NIM811 and SCY-635), which neutralize PPIase activity, but which are not immunosuppressive, also block HCV replication (summarized in **Fig. 2**) is consistent with this hypothesis. In *Drosophila melanogaster*, the CypA homolog, called NinaA, forms a stable and specific complex with the Rh1 isoform of rhodopsin. The formation of this complex is essential for the transit of the visual pigment through the endoplasmic reticulum.[72,73] An elegant study by Schmid and colleagues[74] showed that a proline serves as a molecular timer in the infection of *Escherichia coli* by the filamentous phage fd. The phage infection is activated by the disassembly of 2 domains of its gene-3 protein, which is located at the phage tip. A proline (Pro213) located in the hinge between the 2 gene-3 protein domains, serves as a timer for the infective state. The timer is switched on by *cis* to *trans* and switched off by the unusually slow *trans* to *cis* isomerization of the Gln212-Pro213 peptide bond. The switching rate and the phage infectivity are determined by the local sequence surrounding Pro213, and can be tuned by mutagenesis.[74] Another hypothesis is that the PPIase activity and the auxiliary polypeptide sequestration function of CypA are required for its function in HCV replication. Indeed, mutagenesis of NinaA failed to identify a mutant, which distinguishes the isomerase from the polypeptide sequestration activity of CypA.[72] Similarly, it has been shown that mutations that disrupt the isomerase activity of CypA also disrupt the capacity of CypA to bind HIV-1 Gag in hepatocytes.[70] This is in accordance with the work of Luban and colleagues,[75] who showed that all mutations that neutralize CypA enzymatic activity also preclude CypA incorporation into HIV-1.

The second important question is how do the Cyp inhibitors block HCV replication? Several models have been proposed to explain how Cyps participate in HCV replication. The original model was that Cyps, by interacting with NS5B, increases the affinity of the polymerase to the viral RNA, and therefore enhances HCV replication.[65,66] In this model, Cyp inhibitors, by binding to the hydrophobic pocket of Cyps (ie, CypA), block the ability of Cyps to interact with NS5B, leading to weaker viral RNA binding and the inability to form a functional RNA replication complex (RC) (**Fig. 4**, Model A). Supporting this hypothesis, Yang and colleagues presented pull-down data suggesting that CypA binds NS5B and that the interaction is prevented by CsA.[68] Moreover, studies showed that amino acid changes may arise in NS5B when the HCV replicon is cultured under Cyp inhibitor selection.[35,69,76–78] If CypA and NS5B interact to facilitate HCV replication, they should colocalize to sites of RNA replication. Because the HCV RC is membrane-associated and viral replication is believed to occur on the cytosolic side of modified cellular membranes, CypA, which is predominantly cytosolic, is ideally localized to interact with the HCV RC. Another model was recently proposed by Tang and colleagues[79] who suggest that CypA is responsible for the recruitment of NS5B into the HCV RC in lipid droplets. They showed that CsA reduces NS5B levels in the RC, but not those of NS5A and NS3[79] (see **Fig. 4**, Model B). Moreover, they showed that the RC association of the NS5B mutant protein from a CsA-resistant

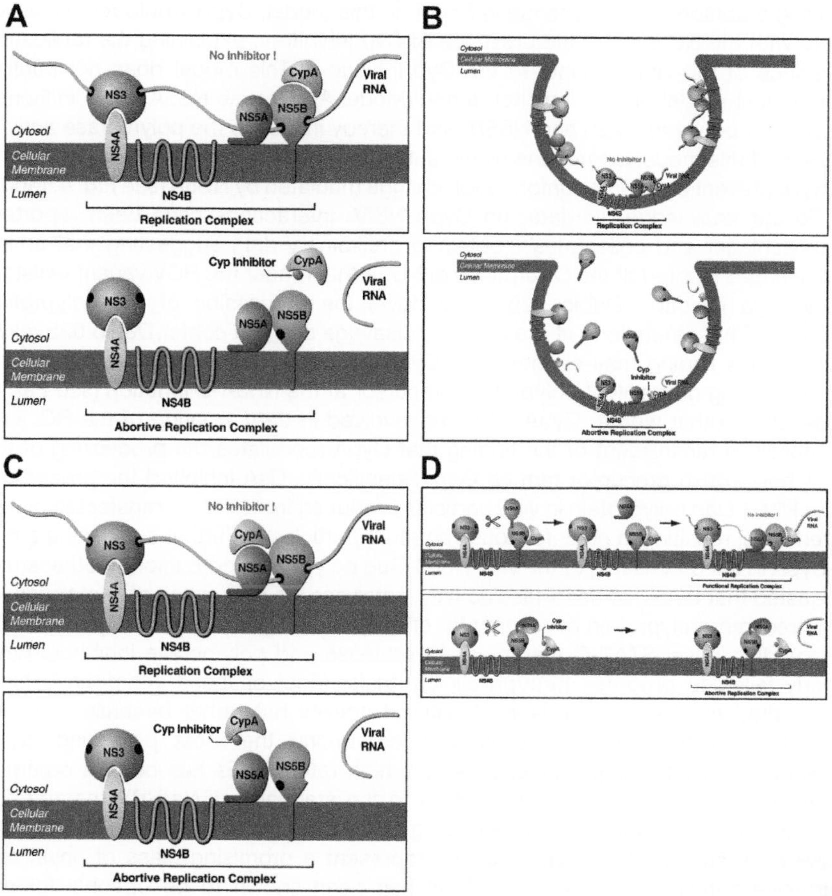

Fig. 4. Mechanisms of anti-HCV action of cyclophilin inhibitors. (*Model A*) Cyp inhibitors block HCV replication by decreasing the affinity of the NS5B polymerase to the viral RNA. (*Model B*) Cyp inhibitors prevent the recruitment of the NS5B polymerase into the RC. (*Model C*) Cyp inhibitors interfere with NS5B-RNA interaction by disrupting the CypA-NS5A interactions. (*Model D*) Cyp inhibitors inhibit HCV replication by hampering the processing of the HCV polyprotein precursor at the NS5A-NS5B junction site.

replicon is not disrupted by CsA.[79] However, they also presented data suggesting that CypA is recruited into the RC by binding to NS5B, and that CsA blocks CypA association with the membrane and with the RC.[79] It is not clear in this model if CypA recruits NS5B into the RC, or the opposite. On the other hand, a growing body of evidence suggests that NS5A might also be implicated in the Cyp inhibitor–mediated block of HCV replication. Specifically, amino acid changes can also occur in NS5A when the HCV replicon is cultured under Cyp inhibitor selection.[35,69,76,78,80,81] Most NS5A mutations conferring resistance to the Cyp inhibitors were mapped into 2 main regions: domain 2 of NS5A, which interacts with NS5B, and the C-terminus of NS5A near the NS5A-NS5B junction. Another attractive model to explain the emergence of mutations in domain 2 of NS5A and the resistance of viral variants to Cyp inhibitors is that the NS5A mutations in the Cyp inhibitor–resistant variants preserve the contact between NS5A and NS5B, but enhance the affinity of NS5B to CypA, possibly by inducing a conformational change in NS5B. In this model, CypA would remain associated with the RC even in the presence of Cyp inhibitors, explaining the replication resistance of the viral variants to the Cyp inhibitors. This model does not conflict with the first model of Cyp inhibitor action (Model A) because NS5A could influence the contact between CypA and NS5B, and thereby influence the polymerase activity of NS5B. If this model is true, one would anticipate that the Cyp inhibitors, by binding to Cyps, prevent the NS5B conformation change mediated by NS5A (see **Fig. 4**, Model C). To our knowledge, to date, no CypA-NS5A interactions have been reported. Bartenschlager and colleagues[69] obtained preliminary data suggesting that amino acid changes located at the C-terminus of NS5A that render the HCV variant resistant to the Cyp inhibitor, Debio 025, slow down the processing of the polyprotein precursor. Thus, mutations at the NS5A-B cleavage site can confer Debio 025 resistance.[69] This finding may suggest that CypA can modulate (decrease or increase) the processing of the HCV polyprotein precursor at the NS5A-B junction (see **Fig. 4**, Model D). In other words, CypA might be involved in the formation of the RC. This hypothesis is reminiscent of the finding that CypA modulates the processing of the HIV-1 polyprotein precursor termed Gag. Specifically, CsA inhibited the processing of the HIV-1 Gag polyprotein in viral particles produced from HIV-1–transfected or –infected cells, resulting in noninfectious immature particles.[82] Further supporting a role for CypA in the processing of the viral HIV-1 Gag polyprotein precursor, another study suggested that CypA, by its PPIase activity, catalyzes the generation of conformers of Gag precursor polyprotein necessary for efficient cleavage by the HIV-1 protease.[83]

Regarding novel STAT-C therapies, 12 protease and polymerase inhibitors have already failed to progress through clinical trials. Most of these compounds have been halted not because of lack of antiviral activity but rather because of unacceptable adverse event (AE) profiles. Even among the most promising drugs currently under later-stage development, a high rate of AEs has been a common observation. The addition of a third drug to the standard pIFNa/RBV therapy has often led to a 2- to 3-fold increase in drug discontinuations. However, several lines of evidence suggest that Cyp inhibitors represent a promising class of novel and alternative anti-HCV agents. First, CypA has been shown to be optional for cell growth and survival. Therefore, its neutralization by Cyp inhibitors should not lead to serious effects in patients. Second, no patient developed a viral breakthrough during treatment with Debio 025, suggesting a high barrier for resistance selection.[39] Third, the AEs mediated by Debio 025 were mild and transient.[39] Further work is needed to determine which activity of Cyps (PPIase, chaperoning, or another unknown activity) controls HCV replication, to understand at a molecular level how this Cyp activity assists HCV replication, and to identify which viral or host proteins are the true Cyp ligands necessary for HCV replication. A complete understanding of the mechanisms that control the antiviral effect of the Cyp inhibitors is imperative because it will not only provide new anti-HCV therapies, but it will also shed light on the early and late steps of the HCV life cycle, which are still poorly understood. Based on the apparent success of the Cyp inhibitor, Debio 025, in phase II studies, it is likely that a second generation of Cyp inhibitors will rapidly emerge. These new Cyp inhibitors will either be derived from CsA like NIM811, Debio 025, and SCY-635, or from other Cyp-neutralizing agents such as sanglifehrins, which bind CypA at sites distinct from the CsA-binding site.[78] A novel sanglifehrin analog called AAE931 exhibited significant anti-HCV activities in vitro.[78] A second generation of Cyp inhibitors should demonstrate increased efficacy and improved safety profiles compared with those of the Cyp inhibitors currently evaluated in the clinic.

SUMMARY

The percentage of patients chronically infected with HCV who reach SVR has profoundly increased since the introduction of plFNa and RBV treatment. However, the current standard plFNa/RBV therapy not only has a low success rate (about 50%), but is often associated with serious side effects. The morbidity and mortality rates associated with HCV are predicted to increase in the coming years, and more efficacious and tolerable therapies are urgently required, particularly for the increasing number of patients who are resistant to plFNa/RBV therapy. Given that there are no approved treatment alternatives available for patients who fail to respond to plFNa/RBV therapy, there is an urgent need for new anti-HCV agents with novel mechanisms of antiviral action. Among the most promising new anti-HCV agents in preclinical and clinical development are the cyclophilin (Cyp) inhibitors. These compounds are a new class of oral inhibitors that suppress HCV replication, most likely by neutralizing the peptidyl-prolyl *cis-trans* isomerase activity of cyclophilins (Cyps).

ACKNOWLEDGMENTS

The authors thank J. Kuhns for secretarial assistance and E. Saphire for CypA structure modeling.

REFERENCES

1. Dienstag JL, McHutchison JG. American Gastroenterological Association technical review on the management of hepatitis C. Gastroenterology 2006;130(1):231–64.
2. Alter MJ. Epidemiology of hepatitis C virus infection. World J Gastroenterol 2007;13(17):2436–41.
3. Soriano V, Madejon A, Vispo E, et al. Emerging drugs for hepatitis C. Expert Opin Emerg Drugs 2008;13(1):1–19.
4. Shepard CW, Finelli L, Alter MJ. Global epidemiology of hepatitis C virus infection. Lancet Infect Dis 2005;5(9):558–67.
5. Davis GL, Balart LA, Schiff ER, et al. Treatment of chronic hepatitis C with recombinant interferon alfa. A multicenter randomized, controlled trial. Hepatitis Interventional Therapy Group. N Engl J Med 1989;321(22):1501–6.
6. Sy T, Jamal MM. Epidemiology of hepatitis C virus (HCV) infection. Int J Med Sci 2006;3(2):41–6.
7. Cross TJ, Antoniades CG, Harrison PM. Current and future management of chronic hepatitis C infection. Postgrad Med J 2008;84(990):172–6.
8. Simmonds P, Bukh J, Combet C, et al. Consensus proposals for a unified system of nomenclature of hepatitis C virus genotypes. Hepatology 2005;42(4):962–73.
9. Manns MP, Wedemeyer H, Cornberg M. Treating viral hepatitis C: efficacy, side effects, and complications. Gut 2006;55(9):1350–9.
10. Davis GL, Albright JE, Cook SF, et al. Projecting future complications of chronic hepatitis C in the United States. Liver Transpl 2003;9(4):331–8.
11. Deuffic-Burban S, Wong JB, Valleron AJ, et al. Comparing the public health burden of chronic hepatitis C and HIV infection in France. J Hepatol 2004;40(2):319–26.
12. World Health Organization. Global surveillance and control of hepatitis C. Report of a WHO consultation organized in collaboration with the viral hepatitis prevention board, Antwerp, Belgium. J Viral Hepat 1999;6(1):35–47.

13. Hoefs J, Aulakh VS. Treatment of chronic HCV infection in special populations. Int J Med Sci 2006;3(2):69–74.
14. Herrine SK, Rossi S, Navarro VJ. Management of patients with chronic hepatitis C infection. Clin Exp Med 2006;6(1):20–6.
15. Shiffman ML, Di Bisceglie AM, Lindsay KL, et al. Hepatitis C antiviral long-term treatment against cirrhosis trial group. Peginterferon alfa-2a and ribavirin in patients with chronic hepatitis C who have failed prior treatment. Gastroenterology 2004;126(4):1015–23.
16. Jeffers LJ, Cassidy W, Howell CD, et al. Peginterferon alfa-2a (40 kd) and ribavirin for black American patients with chronic HCV genotype 1. Hepatology 2004;39(6):1702–8.
17. Muir AJ, Bornstein JD, Killenberg PG, et al. Peginterferon alfa-2b and ribavirin for the treatment of chronic hepatitis C in blacks and non-Hispanic whites. N Engl J Med 2004;350(22):2265–7.
18. Torriani FJ, Rodriguez-Torres M, Rockstroh JK, et al. Peginterferon Alfa-2a plus ribavirin for chronic hepatitis C virus infection in HIV-infected patients. N Engl J Med 2004;351(5):438–50.
19. Carrat F, Bani-Sadr F, Pol S, et al. Pegylated interferon alfa-2b vs standard interferon alfa-2b, plus ribavirin, for chronic hepatitis C in HIV-infected patients: a randomized controlled trial. JAMA 2004;292(23):2839–48.
20. McHutchison JG, Gordon SC, Schiff ER, et al. Interferon alfa-2b alone or in combination with ribavirin as initial treatment for chronic hepatitis C. Hepatitis interventional therapy group. N Engl J Med 1998;339(21):1485–92.
21. Lindsay KL, Trepo C, Heintges T, et al. A randomized, double-blind trial comparing pegylated interferon alfa-2b to interferon alfa-2b as initial treatment for chronic hepatitis C. Hepatology 2001;34(2):395–403.
22. Manns MP, McHutchison JG, Gordon SC, et al. Peginterferon alfa-2b plus ribavirin compared with interferon alfa-2b plus ribavirin for initial treatment of chronic hepatitis C: a randomised trial. Lancet 2001;358(9286):958–65.
23. Fried MW, Shiffman ML, Reddy KR, et al. Peginterferon alfa-2a plus ribavirin for chronic hepatitis C virus infection. N Engl J Med 2002;347(13):975–82.
24. Parfieniuk A, Jaroszewicz J, Flisiak R. Specifically targeted antiviral therapy for hepatitis C virus. World J Gastroenterol 2007;13(43):5673–81.
25. Manns MP, Foster GR, Rockstroh JK, et al. The way forward in HCV treatment – finding the right path. Nat Rev Drug Discov 2007;6(12):991–1000.
26. Goto K, Watashi K, Murata T, et al. Evaluation of the anti-hepatitis C virus effects of cyclophilin inhibitors, cyclosporin A, and NIM811. Biochem Biophys Res Commun 2006;343(3):879–84.
27. Ishii N, Watashi K, Hishiki T, et al. Diverse effects of cyclosporine on hepatitis C virus strain replication. J Virol 2006;80(9):4510–20.
28. Ma S, Boerner JE, TiongYip C, et al. NIM811, a cyclophilin inhibitor, exhibits potent in vitro activity against hepatitis C virus alone or in combination with alpha interferon. Antimicrob Agents Chemother 2006;50(9):2976–82.
29. Nakagawa M, Sakamoto N, Enomoto N, et al. Specific inhibition of hepatitis C virus replication by cyclosporin A. Biochem Biophys Res Commun 2004;313(1):42–7.
30. Watashi K, Hijikata M, Hosaka M, et al. Cyclosporin A suppresses replication of hepatitis C virus genome in cultured hepatocytes. Hepatology 2003;38(5):1282–8.
31. Akiyama H, Yoshinaga H, Tanaka T, et al. Effects of cyclosporin A on hepatitis C virus infection in bone marrow transplant patients. Bone Marrow Transplant 1997;20(11):993–5.

32. Inoue K, Sekiyama K, Yamada M, et al. Combined interferon alpha2b and cyclosporin A in the treatment of chronic hepatitis C: controlled trial. J Gastroenterol 2003;38(6):567–72.
33. Inoue K, Yoshiba M. Interferon combined with cyclosporine treatment as an effective countermeasure against hepatitis C virus recurrence in liver transplant patients with end-stage hepatitis C virus related disease. Transplant Proc 2005; 37(2):1233–4.
34. Coelmont L, Kaptein S, Paeshuyse J, et al. Debio 025, a cyclophilin binding molecule, is highly efficient in clearing HCV replicon containing cells, alone or when combined with specifically targeted antiviral therapy for HCV (STAT-C) inhibitors. Antimicrob Agents Chemother 2009 Mar;53(3):967–76 [epub ahead of print].
35. Hopkins S, Scorneaux B, Huang Z, et al. The Genetic and Biochemical Basis for Resistance to SCY-635 [abstract]. 59th Annual Meeting of the American Association for the Study of Liver Diseases; San Francisco, October 31-November 4, 2008.
36. Mathy JE, Ma S, Compton T, et al. Combinations of cyclophilin inhibitor NIM811 with hepatitis C virus NS3-4A protease or NS5B polymerase inhibitors enhance antiviral activity and suppress the emergence of resistance. Antimicrob Agents Chemother 2008;52(9):3267–75.
37. Paeshuyse J, Kaul A, De Clercq E, et al. The non-immunosuppressive cyclosporin DEBIO 025 is a potent inhibitor of hepatitis C virus replication in vitro. Hepatology 2006;43(4):761–70.
38. Inoue K, Umehara T, Ruegg UT, et al. Evaluation of a cyclophilin inhibitor in hepatitis C virus-infected chimeric mice in vivo. Hepatology 2007;45(4):921–8.
39. Flisiak R, Horban A, Gallay P, et al. The cyclophilin inhibitor Debio 025 shows potent anti-hepatitis C effect in patients coinfected with hepatitis C and human immunodeficiency virus. Hepatology 2008;47(3):817–26.
40. Flisiak R, Feinman SV, Jablkowski M, et al. Efficacy and safety of increasing doses of the cyclophilin inhibitor Debio 025 in combination with pegylated interferon alpha-2a in treatment naive chronic HCV patients. 43rd Annual Meeting of the European Association for the Study of the Liver (EASL 2008). Milan, April 23 – 27, 2008.
41. Hiestand PC, Gräber M, Hurtenbach U, et al. The new cyclosporine derivative, SDZ IMM 125: in vitro and in vivo pharmacologic effects. Transplant Proc 1992; 24(4 Suppl 2):31–8.
42. Rosenwirth B, Billich A, Datema R, et al. Inhibition of human immunodeficiency virus type 1 replication by SDZ NIM 811, a nonimmunosuppressive cyclosporine analog. Antimicrob Agents Chemother 1994;38(8):1763–72.
43. Houck DR, Hopkins S. Preclinical evaluation of SCY-635, a cyclophilin inhibitor with potent anti-HCV activity [abstract]. Hepatology 2006;44(4 Suppl 1):934.
44. Borel JF. History of the discovery of cyclosporin and of its early pharmacological development. Wien Klin Wochenschr 2002;114(12):433–7.
45. Flechner SM. Cyclosporine: a new and promising immunosuppressive agent. Urol Clin North Am 1983;10(2):263–75.
46. Handschumacher RE, Harding MW, Rice J, et al. Cyclophilin: a specific cytosolic binding protein for cyclosporin A. Science 1984;226(4674):544–7.
47. Fischer G, Bang H, Berger E, et al. Conformational specificity of chymotrypsin toward proline-containing substrates. Biochim Biophys Acta 1984;791(1): 87–97.
48. Lang K, Schmid FX, Fischer G. Catalysis of protein folding by prolyl isomerase. Nature 1987;329(6136):268–70.

49. Schiene C, Fischer G. Enzymes that catalyse the restructuring of proteins. Curr Opin Struct Biol 2000;10(1):40–5.
50. Hübner D, Drakenberg T, Forsén S, et al. Peptidyl-prolyl cis-trans isomerase activity as studied by dynamic proton NMR spectroscopy. FEBS Lett 1991; 284(1):79–81.
51. Bang H, Fischer G. Slow conformational changes in protein folding can be accelerated by enzymes. Biomed Biochim Acta 1991;50(10–11):S137–42.
52. Fischer G, Wittmann-Liebold B, Lang K, et al. Cyclophilin and peptidyl-prolyl cis-trans isomerase are probably identical proteins. Nature 1989;337(6206):476–8.
53. Ke HM, Zydowsky LD, Liu J, et al. Crystal structure of recombinant human T-cell cyclophilin A at 2.5 A resolution. Proc Natl Acad Sci U S A 1991;88(21):9483–7.
54. Zydowsky LD, Etzkorn FA, Chang HY, et al. Active site mutants of human cyclophilin A separate peptidyl-prolyl isomerase activity from cyclosporin A binding and calcineurin inhibition. Protein Sci 1992;1(9):1092–9.
55. Wang P, Heitman J. The cyclophilins. Genome Biol 2005;6(7):226 [epub ahead of print].
56. Fruman DA, Burakoff SJ, Bierer BE. Immunophilins in protein folding and immunosuppression. FASEB J 1994;8(6):391–400.
57. Colgan J, Asmal M, Yu B, et al. Cyclophilin A-deficient mice are resistant to immunosuppression by cyclosporine. J Immunol 2005;174(10):6030–8.
58. Braaten D, Luban J. Cyclophilin A regulates HIV-1 infectivity, as demonstrated by gene targeting in human T cells. EMBO J 2001;20(6):1300–9.
59. Cullen BR, Heitman J. Human immunodeficiency virus. Chaperoning a pathogen. Nature 1994;372(6504):319–20.
60. Luban J, Bossolt KL, Franke EK, et al. Human immunodeficiency virus type 1 Gag protein binds to cyclophilins A and B. Cell 1993;73(6):1067–78.
61. Thali M, Bukovsky A, Kondo E, et al. Functional association of cyclophilin A with HIV-1 virions. Nature 1994;372(6504):363–5.
62. Franke EK, Yuan HE, Luban J. Specific incorporation of cyclophilin A into HIV-1 virions. Nature 1994;372(6504):359–62.
63. Liu S, Asparuhova M, Brondani V, et al. Inhibition of HIV-1 multiplication by antisense U7 snRNAs and siRNAs targeting cyclophilin. Nucleic Acids Res 2004; 32(12):3752–9.
64. Sokolskaja E, Sayah DM, Luban J. Target cell cyclophilin A modulates human immunodeficiency virus type 1 infectivity. J Virol 2004;78(23):12800–8.
65. Watashi K, Ishii N, Hijikata M, et al. Cyclophilin B is a functional regulator of hepatitis C virus RNA polymerase. Mol Cell 2005;19(1):111–22.
66. Rice CM, You S. Treating hepatitis C: can you teach old dogs new tricks? Hepatology 2005;42(6):1455–8.
67. Nakagawa M, Sakamoto N, Tanabe Y, et al. Suppression of hepatitis C virus replication by cyclosporin a is mediated by blockade of cyclophilins. Gastroenterology 2005;129(3):1031–41.
68. Yang F, Robotham JM, Nelson HB, et al. Cyclophilin A is an essential cofactor for hepatitis C virus infection and the principal mediator of cyclosporine resistance in vitro. J Virol 2008;82(11):5269–78.
69. Kaul A, Stauffer S, Schmitt J, et al. Role of cyclophilins in hepatitis C virus replication [abstract]. 15th International Symposium on Hepatitis C Virus & Related Viruses. San Antonio (TX), October 5–9, 2008.
70. Bobardt M, Tang H, Sakamoto, et al. The isomerase activity of cyclophilin A is critical for HCV replication [abstract]. 15th International Symposium on Hepatitis C Virus & Related Viruses. San Antonio (TX), October 5–9, 2008.

71. Fischer G, Wawra S. Polypeptide binding proteins: what remains to be discovered? Mol Microbiol 2006;61(6):1388–96.
72. Colley NJ, Baker EK, Stamnes MA, et al. The cyclophilin homolog ninaA is required in the secretory pathway. Cell 1991;67(2):255–63.
73. Stamnes MA, Shieh BH, Chuman L, et al. The cyclophilin homolog ninaA is a tissue-specific integral membrane protein required for the proper synthesis of a subset of *Drosophila* rhodopsins. Cell 1991;65(2):219–27.
74. Eckert B, Martin A, Balbach J, et al. Prolyl isomerization as a molecular timer in phage infection. Nat Struct Mol Biol 2005;12(7):619–23.
75. Braaten D, Ansari H, Luban J. The hydrophobic pocket of cyclophilin is the binding site for the human immunodeficiency virus type 1 Gag polyprotein. J Virol 1997;71(3):2107–13.
76. Fernandes F, Poole DS, Hoover S, et al. Sensitivity of hepatitis C virus to cyclosporine A depends on nonstructural proteins NS5A and NS5B. Hepatology 2007;46(4):1026–33.
77. Robida JM, Nelson HB, Liu Z, et al. Characterization of hepatitis C virus subgenomic replicon resistance to cyclosporine in vitro. J Virol 2007;81(11):5829–40.
78. Wiedmann B, Puyang X, Poulin D, et al. Characterization of mechanism of resistance to cyclophilin inhibitors in HCV replicon [abstract]. 15th International Symposium on Hepatitis C Virus & Related Viruses; San Antonio (TX), October 5–9, 2008.
79. Liu Z, Robotham J, Tang H. Cyclosporine A inhibits cyclophilin A-mediated incorporation of NS5B into HCV replication complex [abstract]. 15th International Symposium on Hepatitis C Virus & Related Viruses, San Antonio (TX), October 5–9, 2008.
80. Goto K, Watashi K, Inoue D, et al. The emergence of a cyclophilin inhibitor-resistant HCV variant with a mutation in NS5A. 14th International Symposium on Hepatitis C Viruses, Glasgow, UK, September 9–13, 2007, P235.
81. Coelmont L, Paeshuyse J, Kaptein S., et al. The cyclophilin inhibitor Debio-025 is a potent inhibitor of hepatitis C virus replication in vitro and has a unique resistance profile. 14th International Symposium on Hepatitis C Viruses, Glasgow, UK, September 9–13, 2007, O61.
82. Streblow DN, Kitabwalla M, Malkovsky M, et al. Cyclophilin A modulates processing of human immunodeficiency virus type 1 p55Gag: mechanism for antiviral effects of cyclosporin A. Virology 1998;245(2):197–202.
83. McCornack MA, Kakalis LT, Caserta C, et al. HIV protease substrate conformation: modulation by cyclophilin A. FEBS Lett 1997;414(1):84–8.

Ribavirin Analogs

William W. Shields, DO[a,*], Paul J. Pockros, MD[b]

KEYWORDS

- Hepatitis C virus • Ribavirin • Anemia • Taribavirin
- Pegylated interferon

Hepatitis C virus (HCV) is the most common bloodborne pathogen in the United States, with 3.2 million persons chronically infected. Approximately 20% of individuals infected will develop cirrhosis during a period of 20 to 30 years, with the potential complications of portal hypertension and its sequelae and hepatocellular carcinoma. Chronic hepatitis C accounts for an estimated 8000 to 10,000 deaths in the United States annually, and this number is expected to more than double by 2010.[1]

Interferon alpha has been the backbone of chronic hepatitis C therapy for the last 20 years.[2] Monotherapy with interferon yields sustained virologic response (SVR) rates of 8% to 17%.[3,4] The use of ribavirin has been investigated as monotherapy in patients with chronic hepatitis C, and it was demonstrated to have improvement in serum aminotransferase levels and histology but had no impact on HCV RNA levels; therefore ribavirin is ineffective when used as a single agent.[5] Subsequent studies showed that ribavirin, in combination with interferon alpha, improved SVR rates up to 36% to 38% compared with standard interferon alone.[6,7] The highest SVR rates are achieved with once-weekly dosing of subcutaneous pegylated interferon combined with daily oral ribavirin, and this is the present standard of care in the United States, European Union, and Japan.[2] Weight-based dosing of ribavirin (1000 mg/d based on weight <75 kg or 1200 mg/d based on weight >75 kg) has been shown to significantly improve SVR rates compared with lower, fixed dosing of ribavirin at 800 mg/d in genotype 1 infection.[8] However, higher dosing of ribavirin is limited by the development of hemolytic anemia, which usually occurs in at least 25% of treated patients.[9] The development of significant anemia often leads to ribavirin dose reductions, which can negatively impact SVR rates.[10]

RIBAVIRIN PHARMACOLOGY

Ribavirin (1-β-D-ribofuranosyl-1H-1,2,4-triazole-3-carboxamide) was first discovered in 1972.[11] Structurally, ribavirin is a purine ribonucleoside analog with broad-spectrum activity against both RNA and DNA viruses (**Fig. 1**).[12] The drug is approved by the US

[a] Department of Gastroenterology and Hepatology, Naval Medical Center San Diego, 34800 Bob Wilson Drive, San Diego, CA 92134, USA
[b] Division of Gastroenterology and Hepatology, Scripps Clinic, The Scripps Research Institute, 10666 North Torrey Pines Road, La Jolla, CA 92037, USA
* Corresponding author.
E-mail address: william.shields@med.navy.mil (W.W. Shields).

Clin Liver Dis 13 (2009) 419–427
doi:10.1016/j.cld.2009.05.006
1089-3261/09/$ – see front matter. Published by Elsevier, Inc.

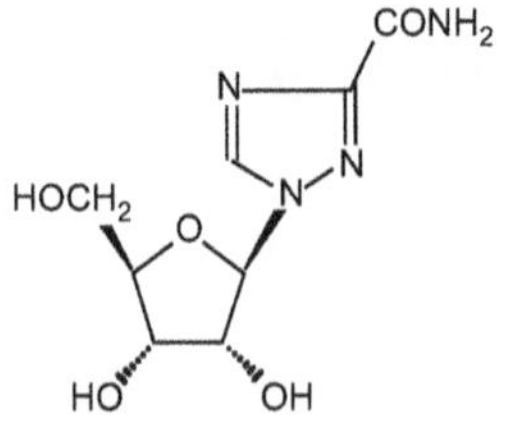

Fig. 1. Chemical structure of ribavirin. (*From* Copegus [ribavirin, USP] [package insert]. Roche Laboratories Inc, Nutley, New Jersey, 2004.)

Food and Drug Administration for the treatment of pediatric respiratory syncytial virus infection and for combination therapy with interferon or pegylated interferon for chronic hepatitis C.[13]

The mechanism of action of ribavirin in chronic hepatitis C is not completely understood. Four mechanisms, indirect and direct, have been proposed (**Fig. 2**).[14] First, ribavirin may be considered a prodrug that enters the cell and is converted to the active metabolites ribavirin-5'-monophosphate (RMP), ribavirin-5'-diphosphate, and ribavirin-5'-triphosphate (RTP) through the sequential action of 3 cellular kinases.[15] RMP mimics inosine-5'-monophosphate and is a competitive inhibitor of host inosine monophosphate dehydrogenase (IMPDH). IMPDH is a required enzyme for the synthesis of guanosine triphosphate (GTP), and GTP is an important substrate for viral

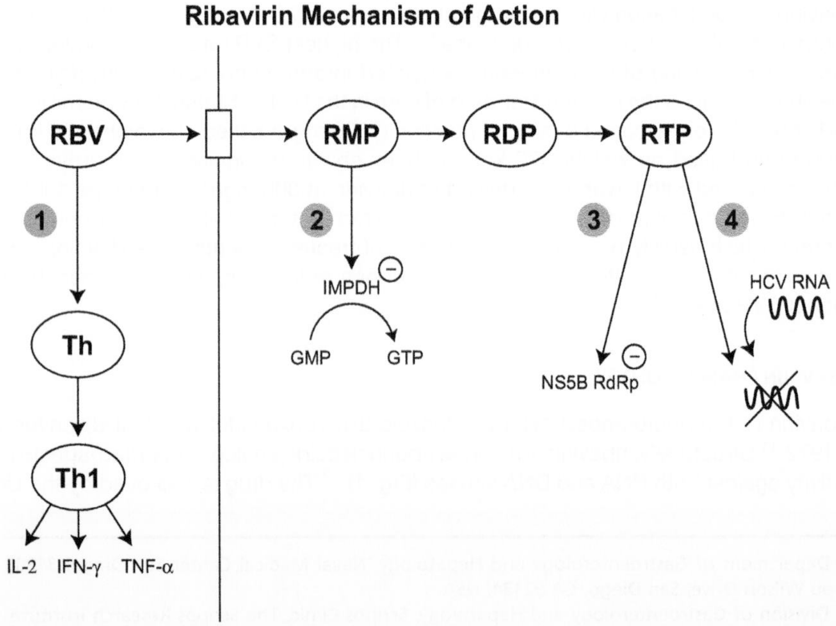

Fig. 2. Proposed mechanisms of action of ribavirin. Ribavirin may act as an immune enhancer by modulating the T-helper cell balance toward Th1 and type 1 cytokines (1). RMP inhibits the host enzyme IMPDH decreasing intracellular levels of GTP (2). RTP may be a direct inhibitor of viral NS5B RdRp (3). RTP may be incorporated into the viral RNA and act as an RNA mutagen (4). (*Data from* Lau JY, Tam RC, Liang TJ, et al. Mechanism of action of ribavirin in the combination treatment of chronic HCV infection. Hepatology 2002;35(5):1002–9).

RNA synthesis. Therefore, inhibition of IMPDH decreases intracellular levels of GTP and may lead to suppression of replication of viral genomes. Second, ribavirin may act to enhance immune clearance of HCV by modulating the T-helper (Th) cell balance toward Th1.[16] Ribavirin augments type 1 cytokines interleukin (IL)-2, interferon-γ, and tumor necrosis factor-α and suppresses type 2 cytokines IL-4 and IL-5.[17] A dominant type 2 cytokine response is associated with the development of chronicity in HCV.[14] Third, ribavirin may have direct antiviral mechanisms through the inhibition of the NS5B RNA dependent RNA polymerase (RdRp). RTP has been shown to have activity against RdRp of bovine viral diarrheal virus, which is closely related to HCV.[14] Lastly, ribavirin may act as an RNA mutagen, as has been shown in a poliovirus model. RTP may be used by the viral RdRp and misincorporated into the viral RNA. RTP can base pair with cytidine and uridine, promoting transitions of A to G and G to A, thus leading to viral "error catastrophe."[18]

The most significant adverse effect of ribavirin is a reversible hemolytic anemia. This effect of ribavirin significantly affects patient quality of life and negatively affects SVR rates. Ribavirin is actively transported into erythrocytes, where it is then converted to its phosphate metabolites. These phosphorylated metabolites cannot diffuse outside of cells, and they progressively accumulate intracellularly during treatment. Increased intracellular ribavirin concentration as phosphorylated metabolites can predict the occurrence of anemia (**Fig. 3**).[19] The increase in phosphorylated metabolites is associated with a marked decrease in cellular ATP levels, leading to a decrease in sodium-potassium pump activity contributing to oxidative damage to the erythrocyte membrane and thus leading to erythrophagocytic extravascular destruction.[20]

RIBAVIRIN ANALOGS

Recent studies of direct antiviral agents have demonstrated that there will continue to be a need for combination of direct antiviral plus pegylated interferon and ribavirin and that deletion of ribavirin from the combination regimen resulted in lowered efficacy.[21,22] Several of these agents promote anemia on their own or worsen ribavirin-associated anemia.[23,24] Therefore, the search for ribavirin analogs, which would have equivalent

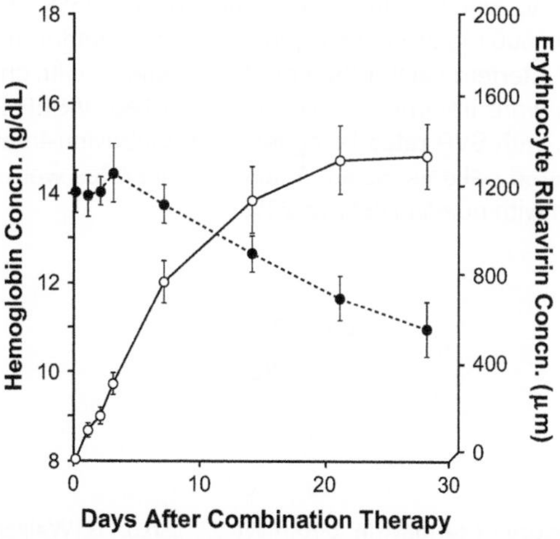

Fig. 3. Intracellular ribavirin concentration predicts the occurrence of anemia. (*From* Homma M, Matsuzaki Y, Inoue Y, et al. Marked elevation of erythrocyte ribavirin levels in interferon and ribavirin-induced anemia. Clin Gastroenterol Hepatol 2004;2:338; with permission).

efficacy, but diminished toxicity, remains an important milestone to HCV treatment. Several compounds have been investigated, as outlined in the following sections.

Taribavirin (Viramidine)

Taribavirin is a 3-carboxamidine derivative of ribavirin. It is a prodrug, which is activated and converted to ribavirin by the enzyme adenosine deaminase (**Fig. 4**).[13] The major site of conversion is in the hepatocyte; therefore this prodrug is able to deliver more ribavirin to the liver and less to other cells, including red blood cells. In turn, this decreases the accumulation of phosphorylated metabolites and subsequent hemolytic anemia. The liver-targeting property of taribavirin has yielded an improved safety profile over ribavirin in animal and human studies.[25] In addition to being a prodrug to ribavirin, taribavirin has been shown to act as a direct inhibitor of nucleoside phosphorylase that slows the degradation of the newly formed active phosphorylated metabolites of ribavirin, which can improve drug efficacy.[26]

The first human studies of taribavirin were reported in 2004. This initial study demonstrated that taribavirin was well tolerated, was rapidly converted to ribavirin, and was renally excreted.[27] A phase 2, open-label study followed, which included 180 patients with chronic hepatitis C. Patients were randomized to receive pegylated interferon alpha-2a 180 μg/wk plus taribavirin (800 mg/d, 1200 mg/d, or 1600 mg/d) or ribavirin (1000 mg/d or 1200 mg/d). The results of this study showed SVR rates of 23%, 37%, and 29% for the 3 arms of taribavirin versus 44% for ribavirin. Significantly fewer patients in the taribavirin arms developed severe anemia, defined as hemoglobin less than 10 g/dL, than in those receiving ribavirin, 4% versus 27%.[28]

The results of this phase 2 study led to 2 large phase 3 clinical trials: viramidine safety and efficacy versus ribavirin (VISER) 1 and VISER 2. VISER 1 compared taribavirin 600 mg twice a day plus pegylated interferon alpha-2b with ribavirin plus pegylated interferon alpha-2b. About 970 patients with chronic hepatitis C, all genotypes, who were treatment-naïve, were enrolled. Overall, SVR rates were lower in those receiving taribavirin (38%) than in those receiving ribavirin (52%). Taribavirin did not meet the criteria for noninferiority to ribavirin efficacy endpoint on an intent-to-treat basis. Taribavirin did demonstrate a superior safety profile, with anemia rates (Hb < 10 g/dL) being significantly lesser than ribavirin (5% vs 24%).[29] VISER 2 compared taribavirin 600 mg twice a day plus pegylated interferon alpha-2a with ribavirin plus pegylated interferon alpha-2a. About 962 patients with chronic hepatitis C of all genotypes, who were treatment-naïve, were enrolled. VISER 2 produced similar results as VISER 1, with SVR rates being lesser in taribavirin-treated patients (40%) than in ribavirin treated patients (55%). Again, anemia rates were significantly lesser with taribavirin than with ribavirin (6% vs 22%).[30]

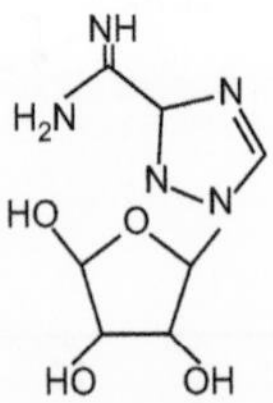

Fig. 4. Chemical structure of taribavirin. (*From* Wu JZ, Larson G, Walker H, et al. Phosphorylation of ribavirin and viramidine by adenosine kinase and cytosolic 5′-nucleotidase II: implications for ribavirin metabolism in erythrocytes. Antimicrob Agents Chemother 2005;49(6):2164–71.)

A post hoc subgroup analysis suggested improved SVR rates with higher weight-based dosing of taribavirin.[31] Therefore, a phase 2b study was initiated in 275 patients with chronic hepatitis C, genotype 1, who were treatment-naïve, that compared taribavirin at doses of 20, 25, or 30 mg/kg/d with weight-based dosing of ribavirin.[32] All patients received pegylated interferon alpha-2b. Interim analysis results at treatment week 24 were presented at the 59th annual meeting of the American Association for the Study of Liver Diseases in 2008. Rapid virologic response rates for the 3 arms of taribavirin were 16.4%, 14.3%, and 16.2% versus 11.4% for ribavirin. The percentage of patients who had undetectable HCV RNA at 12 weeks was 41.8%, 41.4%, and 25% for the 3 arms of taribavirin versus 31.4% for ribavirin. Rates of anemia, defined as hemoglobin less than 10 g/dL, were significantly lower in the taribavirin arms (13.4%, 11.4%, and 19.1%) than for ribavirin (30%). The most common adverse effects were fatigue, headache, nausea, and diarrhea and were similar across all study arms with the exception of diarrhea, which occurs more frequently with taribavirin. This study is ongoing, and further interim results, including end-of-treatment data, have been released by Valeant Pharmaceuticals International, California, USA. The rates of undetectable HCV RNA at 48 weeks (end-of-treatment response) were reported as 43.4%, 32.9%, and 29.4% for the 3 arms of taribavirin versus 32.9% for ribavirin. Rates of anemia at end of treatment were 13.4%, 15.7%, and 27.9% for taribavirin and 32.9% for ribavirin.[33]

Levovirin (ICN 17,621)

Levovirin (1-β-L-ribofuranosyl-1,2,4-triazole-3-carboxamide) is an L-isomer of ribavirin (**Fig. 5**). Similar to ribavirin, levovirin has been shown to enhance Th1 host immune response, which is important in the clearance of HCV infection. Levovirin is not recognized by host kinases, therefore, phosphorylated metabolites do not accumulate. Inhibition of IMPDH has not been demonstrated, and the compound does not accumulate in erythrocytes. Therefore, hemolytic anemia does not occur in normal or HCV-infected persons given this compound. Levovirin has been shown to decrease serum alanine transaminase levels in a murine hepatitis model.[34,35] One large randomized, double-blind, phase 2 clinical trial involving levovirin has been presented;[36] however, the data have not been published in manuscript form. The study showed that although there was a marked reduction in anemia, there was no added benefit in achieving a complete early virologic response when levovirin was combined with pegylated interferon and compared with pegylated interferon monotherapy, and thus the drug was not carried into further trials.

OTHER IMPDH INHIBITORS

VX-497 (Merimepodib)

VX-497 is a phenyloxazole derivative with the chemical name (S)-*N*-3-[3-(3-methoxy-4-oxazol-5-yl-phenyl)-ureido]-benzyl-carbamic acid tetrahydroguran-3-yl-ester (**Fig. 6**).

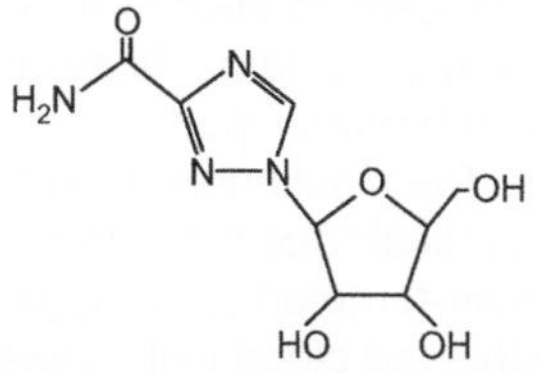

Fig. 5. Chemical structure of levovirin.

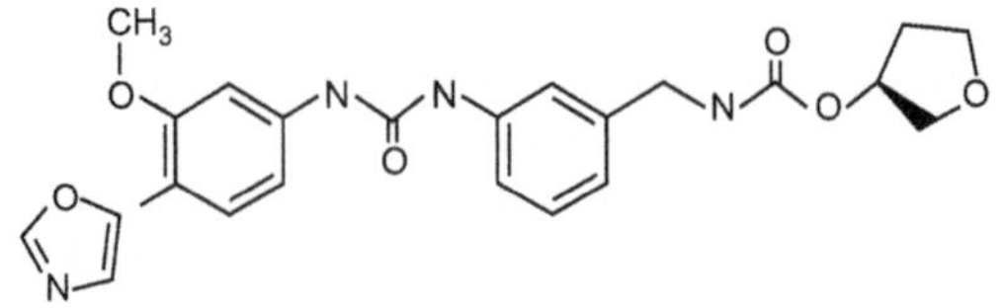

Fig. 6. Chemical structure of VX-497.

VX-497 is a selective, potent, reversible, uncompetitive inhibitor of IMPDH. Early preclinical studies showed that VX-497 demonstrated activity against a variety of viruses and was 10- to 100-fold more potent than ribavirin against hepatits B virus, human cytomegalovirus, respiratory syncytial virus, herpes simplex virus -1, encephalomyocarditis virus, parainfluenza 3 virus, and Venezuelan equine encephalomyelitis virus. There was an additive antiviral effect when combined with interferon alpha.[37] A dose escalation and tolerability study of 55 patients with chronic hepatitis C, who were genotype 1 and treatment-naïve, demonstrated that VX-497 was well tolerated and effective against HCV. In this trial, patients were randomized to standard interferon 3 million IU subcutaneously 3 times a week in combination with VX-497 100 mg or 300 mg every 8 hours for 4 weeks or standard interferon alone. A per protocol analysis showed that standard interferon plus VX-497 100 mg significantly decreased HCV RNA levels compared with standard interferon alone (−1.768 log versus −0.86 log).[38] A second phase 2 study investigated the addition of VX-497 to pegylated interferon alpha-2b and ribavirin in patients with chronic hepatitis C who were nonresponders to previous therapy. In this study, all patients received pegylated interferon alpha-2b and ribavirin, but they were randomized to placebo or VX-497 at 25 mg every 12 hours or 50 mg every 12 hours. At week 24, 8 of 11 patients in the 50-mg group had undetectable HCV RNA, 2 of 10 in the 25-mg group, and 3 of 10 in the placebo group. In general, VX-497 was well tolerated.[39] The final results of this phase 2 trial are pending publication. Further drug development is unlikely in view of recent evidence that ribavirin's antiviral activity is not related to IMPDH inhibition.[40]

Mycophenolate Mofetil

Mycophenolate mofetil(MMF, CellCept) is a potent IMPDH inhibitor. This well-known immunosuppressant compound is used for management after organ transplantation. Because of its IMPDH inhibition, MMF has been studied in combination with interferon alpha. It has been shown to inhibit HCV replication; however, it has been ineffective in improving virologic response rates.[41,42] Because of its immunosuppressive effects, MMF may play a role in the treatment of HCV-related autoimmune diseases.[43]

SUMMARY

Ribavirin is ineffective as monotherapy against HCV; however, it has been shown to be critical in attaining early virologic response and SVR when combined with interferon and/or pegylated interferon. The recent addition of direct antiviral agents to combination therapy will not change this paradigm. Ribavirin has dose-limiting toxicities (primarily hemolytic anemia), which often lead to discontinuation or dose reduction, negatively impacting SVR rates. The mechanism by which ribavirin exerts its antiviral activity remains unknown, but it is likely due to the induction of viral mutagenesis. The ribavirin analog taribavirin is a liver-targeted prodrug, which has less accumulation of phosphorylated metabolites within red blood cells, thereby reducing the incidence of hemolytic anemia. Early studies, which demonstrated equal efficacy with lesser anemia, were encouraging; however, 2 large phase 3 studies were disappointing, because they demonstrated inferiority to ribavirin. A subsequent ongoing phase 2 study, using higher, weight-based dosing of taribavirin, has thus far yielded encouraging results and maintained a significantly less rate of anemia. Taribavirin may be a promising alternative to ribavirin in the future. Other ribavirin analogs and IMPDH inhibitors have yielded less promising results and are not in advanced clinical development.

REFERENCES

1. The Department of Health and Human Services Center for Disease Control and Prevention. Hepatitis C. Available at: http://www.cdc.gov/hepatitis/HCV.htm. Accessed October 9, 2008.
2. National Institutes of Health. Consensus Development Conference Statement: management of hepatitis C. Hepatology 2002;36(5 Suppl. 1):S3–20.
3. Thevenot T, Regimbeau C, Ratziu V, et al. Meta-analysis of interferon randomized trials in the treatment of viral hepatitis C in naïve patients: 1999 update. J Viral Hepat 2001;8(1):48–62.
4. Carithers RL Jr, Emerson SS. Therapy of hepatitis C: meta-analysis of interferon alfa-2b trials. Hepatology 1997;26(3 Suppl. 1):83S–8S.
5. Di Bisceglie A, Conjeevaram HS, Fried MW, et al. Ribavirin as therapy of chronic hepatitis C: a randomized, double-blind, placebo-controlled trial. Ann Intern Med 1995;123(12):897–903.
6. Reichard O, Norkrans G, Frydén A, et al. Randomised, double-blind, placebo-controlled trial of interferon alpha-2b with and without ribavirin for chronic hepatitis C. Lancet 1998;351:83–7.
7. McHutchison JG, Gordon SC, Schiff ER, et al. Interferon alfa-2b alone or in combination with ribavirin as initial treatment for chronic hepatitis C Hepatitis Interventional Therapy Group. N Engl J Med 1998;339(21):1485–92.
8. Hadziyannis SJ, Sette H, Morgan TR, et al. Peginterferon alpha-2a and ribavirin combination therapy in chronic hepatitis C: a randomized study of treatment duration and ribavirin dose. Ann Intern Med 2004;140(5):346–55.
9. Fried MW, Shiffman ML, Reddy KR, et al. Peginterferon alfa-2a plus ribavirin for chronic hepatitis C infection. N Engl J Med 2002;347(13):975–82.
10. Reddy KR, Shiffman ML, Morgan TR, et al. Impact of ribavirin dose reductions in hepatitis C virus genotype 1 patients completing peginterferon alfa-2a/ribavirin treatment. Clin Gastroenterol Hepatol 2007;5(1):124–9.
11. Witkowski JT, Robins RK, Sidwell R, et al. Design, synthesis, and broad spectrum antiviral activity of 1-β-D-ribofuranosyl-1H-1,2,4-triazole-3-carboxamide and related nucleosides. J Med Chem 1972;15(11):1150–4.
12. Copegus (ribavirin, USP) [package insert]. Roche Laboratories Inc, Nutley, New Jersey. 2004.
13. Wu JZ, Larson G, Walker H, et al. Phosphorylation of ribavirin and viramidine by adenosine kinase and cytosolic 5'-nucleotidase II: implications for ribavirin metabolism in erythrocytes. Antimicrob Agents Chemother 2005;49(6):2164–71.
14. Lau JY, Tam RC, Liang TJ, et al. Mechanism of action of ribavirin in the combination treatment of chronic HCV infection. Hepatology 2002;35(5):1002–9.
15. Wu JZ, Walker H, Lau JY, et al. Activation and deactivation of a broad-spectrum antiviral drug by a single enzyme: adenosine deaminase catalyzes two consecutive deamination reactions. Antimicrob Agents Chemother 2003; 47(1):426–31.

16. Shiina M, Kobayashi K, Satoh H, et al. Ribavirin upregulates interleukin-12 receptor and induces T-cell differentiation towards type 1 in chronic hepatitis C. J Gastroenterol Hepatol 2004;19:558–64.
17. Tam RC, Pai B, Bard J, et al. Ribavirin polarizes human T cell responses towards a type 1 cytokine profile. J Hepatol 1999;30(3):376–82.
18. Crotty S, Maag D, Arnold JJ, et al. The broad-spectrum antiviral ribonucleoside ribavirin is an RNA virus mutagen. Nat Med 2000;6(12):1375–9.
19. Homma M, Matsuzaki Y, Inoue Y, et al. Marked elevation of erythrocyte ribavirin levels in interferon and ribavirin-induced anemia. Clin Gastroenterol Hepatol 2004;2(4):337–9.
20. De Franceschi L, Fattovich G, Turrini F, et al. Hemolytic anemia induced by ribavirin therapy in patients with chronic hepatitis C virus infection: role of membrane oxidation damage. Hepatology 2000;31(4):997–1004.
21. Pockros PJ, Balart LA. Advances in hepatology research. Rev Gastroenterol Disord 2008;8(3):194–212.
22. Zeuzem S, Hezode C, Ferenci P, et al. Telaprevir in combination with peginterferon alfa-2a with or without ribavirin in the treatment of chronic hepatitis C: final results of the PROVE 2 study [abstract]. Hepatology 2008;48(Suppl):418A.
23. Pockros PJ, Nelson D, Godofsky E, et al. R1626 plus peginterferon alfa-2a provides potent suppression of hepatitis C virus RNA and significant antiviral synergy in combination with ribavirin. Hepatology 2008;48(2):385–97.
24. Kwo P, Lawitz EJ, McCone J, et al. HCV SPRINT-1: bocepravir plus peginterferon alfa-2b/ribavirin for treatment of genotype 1 chronic hepatitis C in previously untreated patients [abstract]. Hepatology 2008;48(Suppl):1027A.
25. Lin C-C, Yeh LT, Vitarella D, et al. Viramidine, a prodrug of ribavirin, shows better liver-targeting properties and safety profiles than ribavirin in animals. Antivir Chem Chemother 2003;14(3):145–52.
26. Wu JZ, Larson G, Hong Z. Dual-action mechanism of viramidine functioning as a prodrug and as a catabolic inhibitor for ribavirin. Antimicrob Agents Chemother 2004;48(10):4006–8.
27. Lin C-C, Philips L, Xu C. Pharmacokinetics and safety of viramidine, a prodrug of ribavirin in healthy volunteers. J Clin Pharmacol 2004;44(3):265–75.
28. Gish RG, Arora S, Rajender Reddy K, et al. Virological response and safety outcomes in therapy-naïve patients treated for chronic hepatitis C with taribavirin or ribavirin in combination with pegylated interferon alfa-2a: a randomized phase 2 study. J Hepatol 2007;47(1):51–9.
29. Behamou Y, Pockros P, Rodriguez-Torres M, et al. The safety and efficacy of viramidine plus PegIFN alfa-2b versus ribavirin plus PegIFN alfa-2b in therapy-naïve patients infected with hepatitis C virus: phase 3 results (VISER 1) [abstract]. J Hepatol 2006; 44:273A.
30. Marcellin P, Lurie Y, Rodriguez-Torres M, et al. The safety and efficacy of taribavirin plus pegylated interferon alfa-2a versus ribavirin plus pegylated interferon alfa-2a in therapy-naïve patients infected with hepatitis C virus: phase 3 results [abstract]. J Hepatol 2007;46:7A.
31. Pockros PJ, Jacobson IM, Bacon BR, et al. Taribavirin exposure analysis from a previous phase 3 trial correlates with phase 2B weight-based dosing interim results [abstract]. Hepatology 2008;48(Suppl):1138A.
32. Lawitz E, Muir A, Poordad F, et al. Treatment week 24 results of weight-based taribavirin versus weight-based ribavirin both with peginterferon alfa-2b in naïve chronic hepatitis C, genotype 1 patients [abstract]. Hepatology 2008; 48(Suppl):433A.

33. Valeant pharmaceutical international, media center, new release. Available at: www.valeant.com. Accessed December 19, 2008.
34. Tam RC, Ramassamy K, Bard J, et al. The ribavirin analog ICN 17261 demonstrates reduced toxicity and antiviral effects with retention of both immunomodulatory activity and reduction of hepatitis-induced serum alanine aminotransferase levels. Antimicrob Agents Chemother 2000;44(5):1276–83.
35. Lin C-C, Luu T, Lourenco D, et al. Absorption, pharmacokinetics and excretion of levovirin in rats, dogs, and cynomolgus monkeys. J Antimicrob Chemother 2003; 51:93–9.
36. Pockros P, Pessoa M, Diago M, et al. Combination of levovirin and pegylated interferon α-2a fails to generate an induction response comparable to ribavirin and pegylated interferon α-2a in patients with CHC [abstract]. Antivir Ther 2004;9:H17 A32.
37. Markland W, McQuaid TJ, Jain J, et al. Broad-spectrum antiviral activity of the IMP dehydrogenase inhibitor VX-497: a comparison with ribavirin and demonstration of antiviral additivity with alpha interferon. Antimicrob Agents Chemother 2000;44(4):859–66.
38. McHutchison JG, Shiffman ML, Cheung RC, et al. A randomized, double-blind, placebo-controlled dose escalation trial of merimepodib (VX-497) and interferon alpha in previous untreated patients with chronic hepatitis C. Antivir Ther 2005; 10(5):635–43.
39. Marcellin P, Horsmans Y, Nevens F, et al. Phase 2 study of the combination of merimepodib with peginterferon alpha-2b and ribavirin in nonresponders to previous therapy for chronic hepatitis C. J Hepatol 2007;47(4):476–83.
40. Hezode C, Bouvier-Aliasi M, Costentini C, et al. Effect of IMPDH inhibition, Merimepobid (MMPD), assessed in combination with ribavirin (RBV), and alone, on HCV replication: implications regarding RBV's mechanism of action [abstract]. Hepatology 2006;44(4 Suppl 1):615A.
41. Cornberg M, Hinrichsen H, Teuber G, et al. Mycophenolate mofetil in combination with recombinant interferon alfa-2a in interferon nonresponder patients with chronic hepatitis C. J Hepatol 2002;37(6):843–7.
42. Henry SD, Metselaar HJ, Lonsdale RC, et al. Mycophenolic acid inhibits hepatitis C virus replication and acts in synergy with cyclosporine A and interferon alpha. Gastroenterology 2006;131(5):1452–62.
43. Ramos-Casals M, Font J. Mycophenolate mofetil in patients with hepatitis C virus infection. Lupus 2005;14(Suppl 1):S64–72.

Boceprevir, an NS3 Protease Inhibitor of HCV

Kenneth Berman, MD, Paul Y. Kwo, MD*

KEYWORDS

• HCV • Interferon • Ribovirin • Protease • Resistance
• Hepatitis C • Stat-C

Hepatitis C virus (HCV), the most common blood-born infection in the United States, is a major cause of chronic liver disease leading to death from liver failure or hepatocellular carcinoma. Hepatitis C is the most common indication for liver transplantation worldwide and is a major cause of the increased incidence of hepatocellular cancer in the United States.[1] The current paradigm for HCV treatment relies on pegylated interferon (PEG-IFN) and ribavirin as agents that enhance endogenous mechanisms for viral clearance and are dependent on host factors. In patients with genotype 1 HCV infection, the type of infection in most patients in the United States, sustained viral response (SVR) rates remain suboptimal, with less than half of genotype 1–infected individuals going on to achieve SVR. This has led to a shift in the investigational focus for treatment of HCV toward specifically targeted antiviral therapy for HCV (STAT-C) agents. Newer data have demonstrated promise for 2 protease inhibitors, SCH 503034 or boceprevir and VX-950 or telaprevir, both of which appear to be able to improve sustained response while shortening duration of therapy. This review focuses on boceprevir and discusses its mechanism of action, effects on HCV, and viral resistance.

The present standard therapy for patients with HCV genotype 1 is combination PEG-IFN and ribavirin for 48 weeks, which in a large United States trial achieved an SVR rate of 40% to 41%.[2,3] Thus, more than half of genotype 1–infected individuals fail to achieve SVR in the United States. In addition to genotype 1 status, other factors that predict treatment failure include African American race, obesity, older age, diabetes, high viral load, and advanced hepatic fibrosis or steatosis. Many of these factors have been reported to impair the immune response generated by interferon.[4] In addition, adverse events including flu-like symptoms, gastrointestinal side effects, and anemia are common, requiring dose reduction in more than a third of patients and drug discontinuation in approximately 10% of patients.[2] Rigorous management of

Department of Medicine, Division of Gastroenterology/Hepatology, Indiana University School of Medicine, 975 West Walnut Street, IB 327, Indianapolis, IN 46202-5121, USA
* Corresponding author.
E-mail address: pkwo@iupui.edu (P.Y. Kwo).

Clin Liver Dis 13 (2009) 429–439
doi:10.1016/j.cld.2009.05.008
liver.theclinics.com
1089-3261/09/$ – see front matter

side effects has been shown to improve sustained response rates, with higher sustained response rates being noted when patients received most of the interferon and ribavirin. In genotype 1 patients, compliance to combination therapy enhances SVR. In 1 report, patients who adhered to 80% or more of the assigned dose of PEG-IFN-α-2a and ribavirin for 80% or more of treatment duration achieved a sustained response rate of 51% to 63% compared with 34% in patients who took 80% or less of the dose of either drug or completed 80% or less of duration of therapy.[5] Similarly, adherence to 60% or more of ribavirin dose (1000 mg/d for patients less than 75 kg and 1200 mg/d for patients more than 75 kg) has been associated with increased SVR.[6] Patients who received 97% or more of their PEG-IFN-α-2a dose and those who adhered to 60% or more of the intended ribavirin dose achieved an SVR of 64% versus 33% for those who took 60% or less of the intended ribavirin dose, and this occurred regardless of whether doses were temporarily reduced, interrupted, or prematurely stopped.

The use of viral kinetics has allowed the refinement of therapy with PEG-IFN and ribavirin to improve SVR, minimize relapse, and shorten treatment in selected individuals. These concepts remain important as the STAT-C molecules are added to PEG-IFN and ribavirin. Rapid virologic response (RVR), defined as undetectable virus at week 4 of treatment, predicts high SVR rates with shorter duration of therapy with PEG-IFN and ribavirin. Complete early virologic response (cEVR), defined as undetectable virus at week 12 of therapy, is also predictive of SVR.[7,8] Lack of EVR (defined as a 2-log drop in viral load at week 12 of treatment) predicts nonresponse with 48 weeks of PEG-IFN and ribavirin. Patients who achieve RVR may be treated for 24 weeks without any change in SVR rates; however, less than 25% of patients with genotype 1 achieve RVR.[9] Patients who fail to achieve EVR are unlikely to sustain response after 48 weeks of treatment and may require longer duration of therapy if they clear virus by week 24 of treatment.[10,11] The less-than-ideal sustained response rate and side-effect profile of standard therapy has prompted investigation into STAT-C agents in an effort to improve SVR and shorten duration of therapy in genotype 1–infected individuals.

The HCV is a single-stranded RNA molecule that is approximately 9600 nucleotides in length.[12] Viral protein synthesis is mediated by an internal ribosome-entry site that binds directly to ribosomes, and RNA is translated into a polyprotein of 3000 amino acids that is proteolytically cleaved into 4 structural and 6 nonstructural (NS) proteins (**Fig. 1**).[13] The structural proteins are used to assemble new viral particles and the NS proteins support viral RNA replication. The NS3/4A is a serine protease (NS3) and

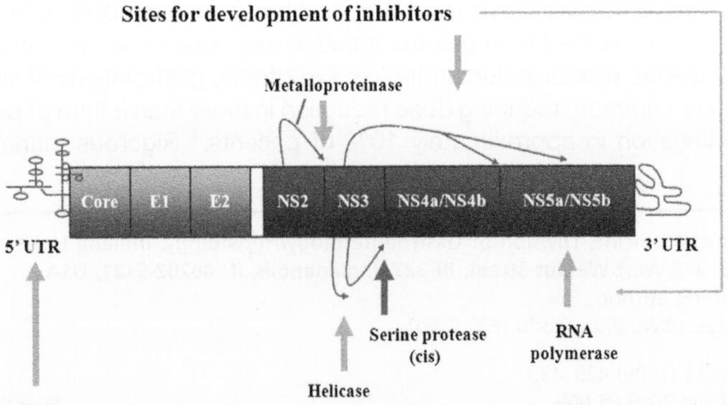

Fig. 1. HCV genome structure and sites for potential STAT-C development.

cofactor (NS 4A) that catalyzes the posttranslational processing of NS proteins from the polyprotein, which is important for viral replication. The NS3 protease cleaves NS4A-NS4B, NS4B-NS5A, and NS5A-NS5B junctions. The products released go on to form a replicative complex responsible for forming viral RNA. Thus, NS3/4A provides an ideal target for antiviral therapy.

HCV replicons have provided an important tool toward the investigation of the serine protease as a potential target for anti-HCV therapies. Before HCV replicons, in vitro HCV replication models had been difficult to establish. In 1999, Lohmann and colleagues[14] described a reliable method of HCV replication with subgenomic HCV RNA in a hepatoma cell line. Based on the finding that in other viral replication models, structural proteins are not required for RNA replication, the HCV RNA genome was modified. Structural proteins were replaced with a selectable marker, in this case, a gene encoding neomycin phosphotransferase (NPT), which inactivates the cytotoxic drug G418. The hepatoma cells were then transfected with the subgenomic RNA replicon and placed in a medium containing G418. Only cells in which the replicon amplified sufficiently were able to produce NPT and confer G418 resistance. The surviving cells were isolated to form colonies of cell clones that carry stable replicating HCV replicons. This technique has allowed evaluation of therapeutic agents that inhibit viral replication and characterization of resistant mutants.[13]

Inhibition of NS3 may have a second therapeutic effect by restoring virally suppressed endogenous interferon pathways. Interferon regulatory factor 3 (IRF-3) is phosphorylated by a virus-activated kinase to induce transcription of interferons and other antiviral genes. As demonstrated by Foy and colleagues,[15] replicating HCV RNA blocks IRF-3 phoshorylation. In this manner, HCV is able to blunt endogenous interferon response. Furthermore, NS3 is the key enzyme responsible for blocking IRF-3 phoshorylation, and cells treated with the NS3 protease inhibitor, SCH6, are able to phosphorylate IRF-3.

In the last decade, drug design targeted at the NS3 protease site has produced multiple protease inhibitors, including BILIN 2061, VX-950, or telaprevir, and SCH 503034, or boceprevir. The protease inhibitor BILIN 2061 provided "proof of concept" data with marked direct antiviral activity; however, further investigation in humans was stopped because of cardiac toxicity in animals.[16,17] Telaprevir and boceprevir have shown early promising data on viral suppression. Boceprevir is a structurally novel peptidomimetic ketoamide HCV NS3 protease inhibitor that binds reversibly to the NS3 active site (**Fig. 2**). Malcolm and colleagues[18] demonstrated a robust antiviral activity of boceprevir on HCV replicons. Treatment of HCV replicons resulted in a 1.5- to 2-log drop in RNA levels at 72 hours and a 3.5- to 4-log drop by day 15 (**Fig. 3**). No toxic hepatocyte effects were seen. Cells treated with boceprevir and

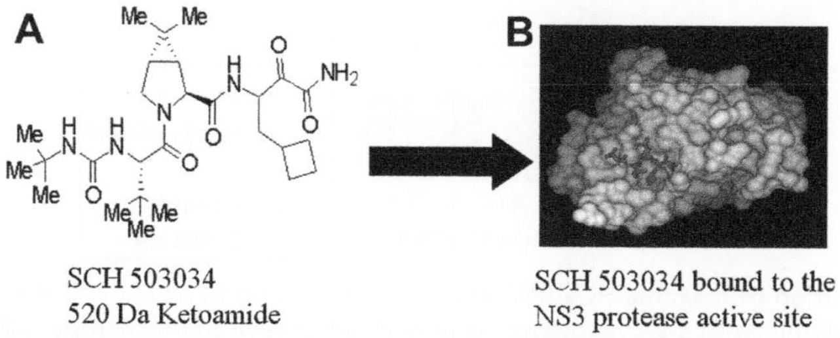

Fig. 2. (*A*) SCH 503034 (boceprevir) structure. (*B*) SCH 503034 (boceprevir) bound to the NS3 protease active site.

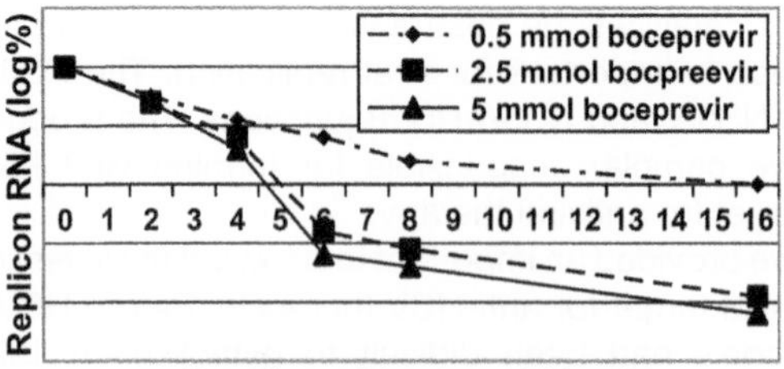

Fig. 3. Effect of treatment duration on HCV replicon RNA treated with 0.5, 2.5, and 5.0 μM SCH 503034. (*Data from* Malcolm BA, Liu R, Lahser F, et al. SCH 503034, a mechanism-based inhibitor of hepatitis C virus NS3 protease, suppresses polyprotein maturation and enhances the antiviral activity of alpha interferon in replicon cells. Antimicrob Agents Chemother 2006;50:1013–20.)

interferon-α had a greater HCV replicon suppression than either agent alone, and this effect appeared to be additive, rather than synergistic. These promising in vitro data allowed boceprevir to enter clinical trials.

The first of these trials was a European phase 1 clinical trial that compared boceprevir monotherapy with PEG-IFN-α-2b monotherapy and PEG-IFN-α-2b plus boceprevir therapy in a nonresponder population.[19] Twenty-six patients with HCV genotype 1a or 1b, who previously did not achieve an EVR with PEG-IFN-α-2b with or without ribavirin, were enrolled and randomized to a 3-way crossover study with 2 doses of boceprevir. Treatment consisted of boceprevir monotherapy (200 or 400 mg 3 times a day) for 1 week, PEG-IFN-α-2b (1.5 μg/kg) weekly for 2 weeks and combination PEG-IFN-α-2b plus boceprevir for 2 weeks. At least 2 weeks between treatments was allowed for washout of the therapies. Combination therapy yielded greater reductions in viral load than either drug given as monotherapy. In the nonresponder patients treated with PEG-IFN-α-2b and boceprevir 200 mg 3 times a day, a maximum mean change in HCV RNA of $-2.28 \pm 1.03 \log_{10}$ was observed. In those treated with PEG-IFN-α-2b and boceprevir 400 mg 3 times a day, a maximum mean change in HCV RNA of $-2.68 \pm 1.12 \log_{10}$ was observed (**Fig. 4**). In the monotherapy arms, single-week therapy with boceprevir 200 or 400 mg only, 3 times daily resulted in viral load reductions of

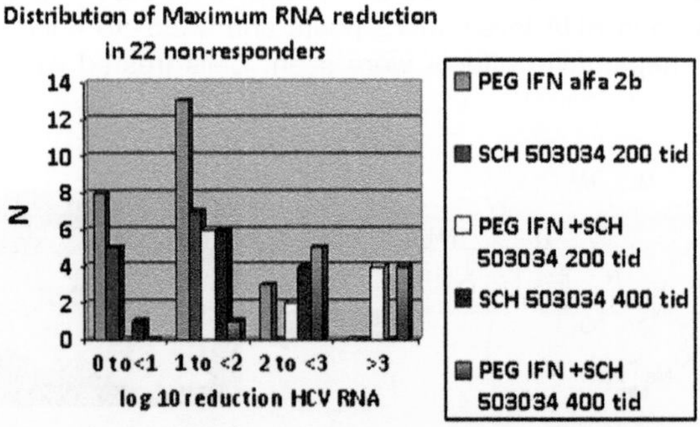

Fig. 4. Distribution of maximal HCV RNA reduction according to treatment. Previous nonresponders randomized to 3-way crossover trial with boceprevir monotherapy (200 or 400 mg 3 times a day) for 1 week, PEG-IFN-α-2b (1.5 μg/kg) weekly for 2 weeks, and combination PEG-IFN-α-2b plus boceprevir for 2 weeks.

$-1.08 \pm 0.22 \log_{10}$ and $-1.61 \pm 0.21 \log_{10}$, respectively. Two-week monotherapy with PEG-IFN-α-2b yielded RNA reductions of -1.08 to $-1.26 \log_{10}$. Four patients did not complete the study, and no new adverse events were seen. Additionally, there was no difference in safety parameters in patients treated with 200 or 400 mg of boceprevir as compared with PEG-IFN-α-2b. Pharmacokinetic phase 1 data did not reveal significant interaction between PEG-IFN-α-2b and boceprevir, with area-under-the-curve values for each drug yielding similar results for monotherapy (boceprevir or PEG-IFN-α-2b) and combination therapy, suggesting little interaction.[19]

With these preliminary data, a phase 2 dose-finding boceprevir study was initiated with several aims, which were to determine what the optimal boceprevir dose was, whether ribavirin is required in combination with PEG-IFN-α-2b and boceprevir, and what the optimal duration would be in a null responder population.[20] In this study, 357 null responders who either failed to achieve EVR or failed to clear virus with more than 12 weeks PEG-IFN-α-2b/ribavirin therapy were enrolled and treated with PEG-IFN-α-2b/ribavirin plus placebo, PEG-IFN-α-2b plus boceprevir in ascending doses (100/200/400/800 mg) 3 times daily or PEG-IFN-α-2b/boceprevir 400 mg 3 times a day plus ribavirin. After an interim analysis by the Data Safety Monitoring Board, the protocol was amended, and all responding patients (defined as less than 10,000IU/mL on original therapy) were assigned to receive PEG-IFN-α-2b, ribavirin, and boceprevir 800 mg 3 times a day for 24 weeks. Although the overall sustained response rate was low, this trial established several important concepts in the treatment of HCV nonresponders with boceprevir. First, for treatment of null responders, ribavirin is required for optimal response in combination with NS3 protease inhibitors such as boceprevir. The optimal boceprevir dose was 800 mg 3 times a day, a dose that no patient initially received. In addition, more rapid time to undetectable HCV RNA and longer duration of therapy with undetectable HCV RNA predicted sustained response The null responders randomized to the PEG-IFN-α-2b/ribavirin without boceprevir arm (control) who demonstrated interferon responsiveness (1–2 log reduction at week 13) were more likely to go on to sustained response with the addition of boceprevir.

These preliminary results led to the design of a phase 2 clinical trial, HCV serine protease inhibitor therapy-1 (SPRINT-1), evaluating boceprevir in combination with PEG-IFN and ribavirin in HCV genotype 1 treatment-naïve patients. Although final results are not yet available, the preliminary data suggest that boceprevir will improve sustained response rates while potentially shortening duration of treatment to 28 weeks. In this multiarm trial, genotype 1 subjects were randomized to receive PEG-IFN-α-2b, weight-based ribavirin, and boceprevir therapy, 800 mg 3 times a day for 28 or 48 weeks, or a lead-in strategy with 4 weeks of PEG-IFN-α-2b and ribavirin followed by boceprevir 800 mg 3 times a day with PEG-IFN-α-2b and ribavirin, and these treatment arms were compared with standard therapy of PEG-IFN-α-2b and ribavirin for 48 weeks (**Fig. 5**). The rationale for the potential benefit of a lead-in strategy is based on the fact that both PEG-IFN-α-2b and ribavirin reach steady-state concentrations by week 4, and with the lead-in strategy, patients have the protease inhibitor added when the backbone drug levels have been optimized and the patient's immune system has been activated. This approach may minimize the period of time when there is a "functional monotherapy" with a direct antiviral, potentially reducing the likelihood for the development of resistance. This strategy may also have the potential to reduce the likelihood of the development of resistance by identifying patients who are responders to interferon and ribavirin before giving them a protease inhibitor or other STAT-C drug.

Interim data, including 12-week SVR (SVR-12), for the 28-week treatment arms with or without lead-in, have been presented.[21] In this multicenter, international trial,

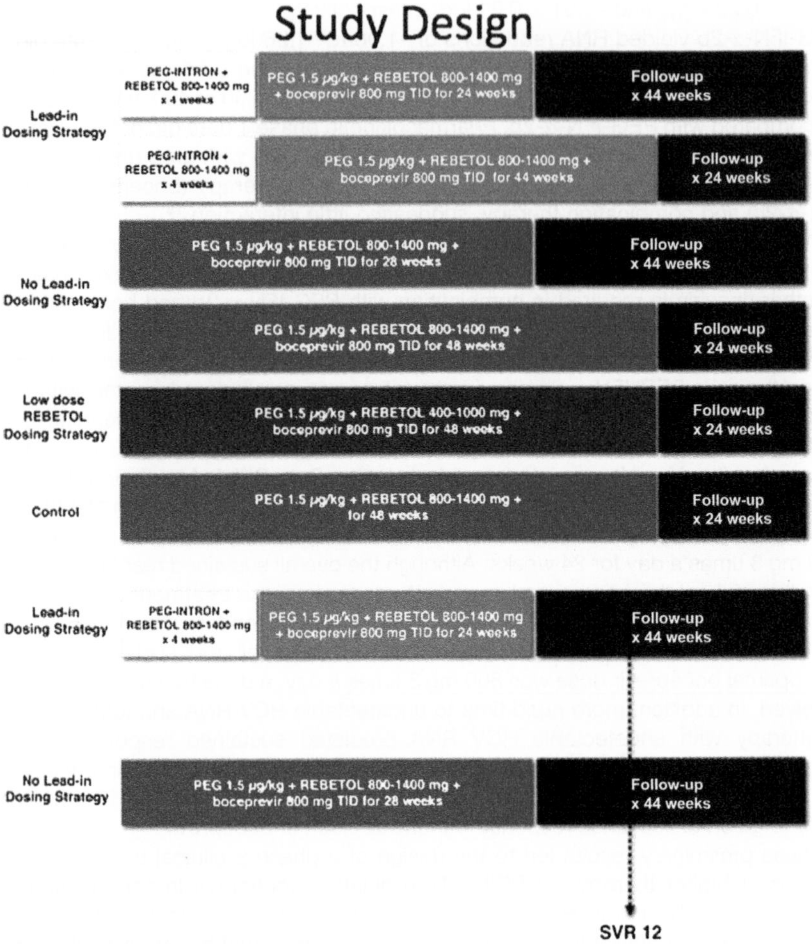

Fig. 5. SPRINT-1 trial treatment arms are shown. Preliminary data from the 28-week treatment arms are available.

approximately 100 subjects were enrolled in each arm and were stratified for the presence of cirrhosis and African American race. The demographic data are shown in **Table 1**. Compared with standard therapy with PEG-IFN-α-2b/ribavirin, significantly more patients in the triple-therapy groups achieved an RVR (62%, 38%, and 8% for PEG-IFN-α-2b/ ribavirin/boceprevir with lead-in, PEG-IFN-α-2b/ ribavirin/boceprevir without lead-in and standard therapy, respectively) and c EVR (79%, 69%, and 34%). In this study, RVR and EVR were defined by the week of boceprevir therapy, thus in the lead-in arm, the week 4 and week 12 RVR and cEVR results were at weeks 8 and 16 of total therapy. Patients with lead-in therapy had higher rates of RVR and EVR; however, the 12-week SVR was similar in these groups at 57% and 55%, respectively (**Fig. 6**). In a subgroup analysis, 44% to 47% of African American patients treated with 28 weeks of triple therapy achieved SVR. Although the number of patients is small (15 and 18 patients respectively), this is a considerable improvement over the 21% to 23% SVR previously reported after 48 weeks of standard therapy with PEG-IFN-α-2b and ribavirin and ribavirin in large United States trials. Regarding

Table 1
Baseline characteristics for patients in 28-week treatment arms of SPRINT-1 trial

	P/R Lead-in → P/R/Boceprevir N = 103[‡]	P/R/Boceprevir N = 107	P/R Control N = 104
Gender Male (%)	50	59	67
Race Caucasian (%)	83	80	80
Mean age (years)	47.7	46.4	48.3
Mean weight (kg)	79.9	83.4	83.4
HCV subtype (%)			
1a	51	63	51
1b	36	28	40
Viral load mean ($\log_{10}$ IU/mL)	6.5	6.6	6.5
HCV RNA >600,000 IU/mL (%)	87	92	90
Cirrhosis (%)	7	7	8

[‡] Boceprevir added to treatment regimen after 4 week lead-in of PEG-IFN α-2b + ribavirin.
Abbreviations: P, pegylated interferon; R, ribavirin.

predictability of PEG-IFN-α-2b/ribavirin/boceprevir, 86% of those who achieved an RVR in the lead-in arm (week 8 of total therapy) went on to SVR-12 after 28 weeks of treatment with triple therapy, and in the non–lead-in arm, 74% of individuals who achieved RVR went on to SVR. Relapse rates were comparable in the 28-week treatment arms at 18% to 19%, the presence of RVR in either arm markedly reducing relapse rates. Treatment discontinuation rates were higher in the triple-therapy groups compared with the standard therapy (26%–28% vs 14%). Adverse events were more common in the boceprevir groups compared with PEG-IFN-α-2b/ribavirin treatment (11%–15% vs 8%) and largely due to anemia and dysgeusia, with no new adverse events noted. Most hemoglobin reductions were grade 1 and 2 (World Health Organization criteria), and no increase in skin or subcutaneous disorders was noted. These

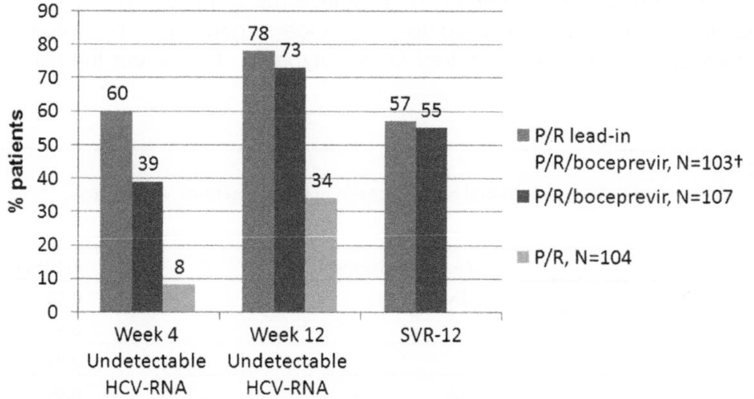

Fig. 6. Preliminary data from SPRINT-1 trial demonstrating RVR, EVR, and 12-week SVR (SVR-12) rates. Patients treated with 28 weeks boceprevir, PEG-IFN-α-2b, and ribavirin with or without lead therapy or PEG-IFN-α-2b and ribavirin.

preliminary results suggested that SVR rates with PEG-IFN, ribavirin, and boceprevir for 28 weeks, regardless of treatment paradigm, appear to be higher than standard of care with PEG-IFN and ribavirin for 48 weeks. The 48-week treatment arm results will better define optimal treatment paradigms for HCV genotype 1 with PEG-IFN-α-2b, ribavirin, and boceprevir.

A major concern with the addition of STAT-C molecules, such as boceprevir, to PEG-IFN and ribavirin, is the development of drug-resistant mutations. In vitro replicon data have demonstrated the emergence of resistant mutations in the presence of STAT-C molecules, and this has been noted with all of the protease inhibitors in development. In vivo, because of the high replication rate and error-prone viral RNA-dependent RNA polymerase, a single host may carry a mixture of HCV viral stains or quasispecies. Resistance has been reported with ribavirin; however, specific resistance to interferon-α is more controversial.[22] In vivo sequencing data have demonstrated the emergence of low- to moderate-level resistant mutations (T54A, V170A, and A156S) and a single high-level mutation (A156T), and these mutations appear to show cross resistance with other protease inhibitors (**Table 2**).[23,24] In the early phase 2 study using lower (nonoptimal dose) doses of boceprevir with varying combinations of PEG-IFN-α -2b and ribavirin, boceprevir resistant mutants were found in most patients not achieving SVR.[25] Ideally, appropriately dosed therapy with boceprevir, PEG-IFN, and ribavirin will allow viral suppression before the emergence or dominance of resistant strains or will allow reduction in replicative fitness, such that the resistant strains will retain sensitivity to PEG-IFN and ribavirin.

Reports of treatment-naïve patients harboring dominant quasispecies resistant to protease inhibitors raise concern about the rapid selection of resistant mutants during STAT-C treatment. Two later studies with more than 1000 HCV genotype 1 patients have described the prevalence of protease inhibitor–resistant strains in treatment-naïve subjects.[26,27] For genotype 1a, the amino acid substitutions associated with decreased sensitivity to NS3 protease inhibitors such as boceprevir (R155K, V36L, V36M, T54S, R109K, and V170A) occurred in 2% to 5% of patients. The R155K mutant has a moderate to high level of resistance to NS3 protease inhibitors, and the remainder of the mutants found carried a low level of resistance to protease inhibitors. Extension of this evaluation to polymerase and protease inhibitors found the prevalence of resistant mutants to genotype 1a to be 8.6%. In contrast, genotype 1b patients had a low prevalence (1.4%) of dominant resistant mutations. This finding is likely a result of a greater barrier to resistance, as 2 nucleotide substitutions to the NS3 domain are required to confer resistance in genotype 1b compared with only 1 nucleotide substitution required for genotype 1a. To prevent the selection of

Table 2
Boceprevir-resistant HCV mutations and prevalence noted in treatment-naïve patients

Mutation	Level of Resistance	Prevalence (%)
V36L	Low	0.56
V36M	Low	0.65
T54S	Low	0.84
R109K	Low	0.09
V170A	Low	0.09
R155K	Moderate to high	0.65

resistant strains, pretreatment resistance screening may be useful to tailor treatment regimens. Moreover, combination STAT-C therapies may provide the ideal treatment by ensuring quick viral suppression that can evade resistant patterns and prevent the generation of new variants.

Newer studies have evaluated the use of combination STAT-C therapy in HCV replicon models.[28] HCV-796 is a nonnucleoside inhibitor of the NS5B polymerase that has previously demonstrated antiviral activity. Clinical trials were halted, however, after patients who received HCV-796 developed elevated liver test levels. Single amino acid mutations near the HCV-796 binding site lead to drug resistance, particularly at the C316Y site. HCV replicons with reduced susceptibility to HCV-796 were treated with boceprevir, and similarly, replicons with reduced susceptibility to boceprevir were treated with HCV-796. Boceprevir susceptibility was not diminished in the mutant replicon with reduced susceptibility to HCV-796, and similarly, HCV-796 susceptibility was not altered by the mutations conferring reduced boceprevir susceptibility. The combination significantly reduced the emergence of resistant colonies; however, replicon cells could be isolated at low drug concentrations. In a similar report, Flint and colleagues[29] applied selective pressures to HCV replicons with combinations of varying doses of boceprevir and HCV-796 to develop dually resistant replicons. Analysis of the resistant replicons demonstrated mutations at NS5B-C316Y (conferring HCV-796 resistance) and NS3-V170A (conferring boceprevir resistance) coexisting in a single genome. Based on replicative capacity compared with a nonmutant parent replicon, the V170A mutation did not alter replicon fitness, whereas the C316Y mutation resulted in diminished fitness. The double mutant (V170A and C316Y) also demonstrated reduced fitness. Similar results were noted by comparing the efficiency of colony formation in the mutant strains. Resistance testing demonstrated susceptibility of these replicons to PEG-IFN-α-2b, and subsequent interferon treatment led to replicon clearance. These data are important, as they demonstrate the ability for HCV quasispecies to become dually resistant to STAT-C drugs of different classes (protease inhibitor and polymerase inhibitor) but to still retain sensitivity to PEG-IFN-α-2b.

Standard therapy for HCV genotype 1 leads to sustained response rates of approximately 40%. The addition of STAT-C molecules to PEG-IFN and ribavirin has been shown to improve the SVR rate in addition to shortening the duration of treatment in genotype 1 individuals. Thus far, the protease inhibitors boceprevir and telaprevir have shown early promise. In vitro and in vivo data have demonstrated viral suppression with boceprevir and superior suppression with boceprevir in combination with PEG-IFN. Early phase 2 studies have established that optimal response to boceprevir depends on ribavirin therapy and PEG-IFN-α-2b responsiveness in nonresponders. Preliminary data from the SPRINT-1 trial are notable for several findings. The study suggests that a lead-in strategy with PEG-IFN/ribavirin therapy may diminish resistance and optimize antiviral response by allowing these drugs to achieve a steady state before a protease inhibitor is added. Twelve-week SVR was 55% to 57% with 28 weeks of therapy, which is superior to standard therapy for 48 weeks. Finally, response rates in African Americans, who typically have poor response to standard therapy, were higher than has been previously reported. As with the resistance seen in the development of HIV therapy, the emergence of resistance to protease inhibitors has been an important consideration. The emergence of drug-resistant mutations suggests that if anti-HCV treatment does not completely suppress replication, selection of resistant HCV strains may occur. However, in vitro data with HCV replicons dually resistant to boceprevir and a first generation polymerase inhibitor have demonstrated successful viral clearance with the addition of PEG-IFN, suggesting a future paradigm to ameliorate the development of resistance. This provides a rationale for future therapies, similar to HIV treatment, with multiple agents used to rapidly suppress viral replication and prevent the emergence of resistant mutations, although in the immediate future, PEG-IFN and ribavirin will remain the backbone of treatment.

REFERENCES

1. Verna EC, Brown RS Jr. Hepatitis C virus and liver transplantation. Clin Liver Dis 2006;10:919–40.
2. Manns MP, McHutchison JG, Gordon SC, et al. Peginterferon alfa-2b plus ribavirin compared with interferon alfa-2b plus ribavirin for initial treatment of chronic hepatitis C: a randomised trial. Lancet 2001;358:958–65.
3. Sulkowski M, Lawitz E, Shiffman ML, et al. Final results of the IDEAL (Individualized Dosing Efficacy Versus Flat Dosing To Assess Optimal Pegylated Interferon Therapy) Phase IIIB Study. J Hepatol 2008;48:S370–1.
4. Zeuzem S. Heterogeneous virologic response rates to interferon-based therapy in patients with chronic hepatitis C: who responds less well? Ann Intern Med 2004; 140:370–81.
5. McHutchison JG, Manns M, Patel K, et al. Adherence to combination therapy enhances sustained response in genotype-1-infected patients with chronic hepatitis C. Gastroenterology 2002;123:1061–9.
6. Reddy KR, Shiffman ML, Morgan TR, et al. Impact of ribavirin dose reductions in hepatitis C virus genotype 1 patients completing peginterferon alfa-2a/ribavirin treatment [see comment]. Clin Gastroenterol Hepatol 2007;5:124–9.
7. Zeuzem S, Buti M, Ferenci P, et al. Efficacy of 24 weeks treatment with peginterferon alfa-2b plus ribavirin in patients with chronic hepatitis C infected with genotype 1 and low pretreatment viremia. [see comment]. J Hepatol 2006;44: 97–103.
8. Ferenci P, Fried MW, Shiffman ML, et al. Predicting sustained virological responses in chronic hepatitis C patients treated with peginterferon alfa-2a (40 KD)/ribavirin. J Hepatol 2005;43:425–33.
9. Jensen DM, Morgan TR, Marcellin P, et al. Early identification of HCV genotype 1 patients responding to 24 weeks peginterferon alpha-2a (40 kd)/ribavirin therapy. [see comment][erratum appears in Hepatology. 2006 Jun;43(6):1410]. Hepatology 2006;43:954–60.
10. Berg T, von Wagner M, Nasser S, et al. Extended treatment duration for hepatitis C virus type 1: comparing 48 versus 72 weeks of peginterferon-alfa-2a plus ribavirin. Gastroenterology 2006;130:1086–97.
11. Pearlman BL, Ehleben C, Saifee S. Treatment extension to 72 weeks of peginterferon and ribavirin in hepatitis C genotype 1-infected slow responders. Hepatology 2007;46:1688–94.
12. Lauer GM, Walker BD. Hepatitis C virus infection. N Engl J Med 2001;345:41–52.
13. Bartenschlager R. Hepatitis C virus replicons: potential role for drug development. Nat Rev Drug Discov 2002;1:911–6.
14. Lohmann V, Korner F, Koch J, et al. Replication of subgenomic hepatitis C virus RNAs in a hepatoma cell line. Science 1999;285:110–3.
15. Foy E, Li K, Wang C, et al. Regulation of interferon regulatory factor-3 by the hepatitis C virus serine protease. Science 2003;300:1145–8.
16. Lamarre D, Anderson PC, Bailey M, et al. An NS3 protease inhibitor with antiviral effects in humans infected with hepatitis C virus. Nature 2003;426:186–9.

17. Hinrichsen H, Benhamou Y, Wedemeyer H, et al. Short-term antiviral efficacy of BILN 2061, a hepatitis C virus serine protease inhibitor, in hepatitis C genotype 1 patients. Gastroenterology 2004;127:1347–55.
18. Malcolm BA, Liu R, Lahser F, et al. SCH 503034, a mechanism-based inhibitor of hepatitis C virus NS3 protease, suppresses polyprotein maturation and enhances the antiviral activity of alpha interferon in replicon cells. Antimicrob Agents Chemother 2006;50:1013–20.
19. Sarrazin C, Rouzier R, Wagner F, et al. SCH 503034, a novel hepatitis C virus protease inhibitor, plus pegylated interferon alpha-2b for genotype 1 nonresponders. [see comment]. Gastroenterology 2007;132:1270–8.
20. Schiff E, Poordad FF, Jacobson IM, et al. Role of interferon response during RE-Treatment of null responders with boceprevir combination therapy: results of phase II trial [abstract]. Gastroenterology 2008;134:A755.
21. Kwo P, Lawitz E, McCone J, et al. Interim results from HCV sprint-1: RVR/EVR from phase 2 study of boceprevir plus pegintrontm (peginterferon alfa-2b)/ribavirin in treatment naive subjects with genotype-1 CHC [abstract]. J Hepatol 2008;48:S372.
22. Young Kung-Chia, Lindsay KL, Lee Ki-Jeong, et al. Identification of a ribavirin-resistant NS5B mutation of hepatitis C virus during ribavirin monotherapy. Hepatology 2003;38:869–78.
23. Zhou Y, Bartels DJ, Hanzelka BL, et al. Phenotypic characterization of resistant Val36 variants of hepatitis C virus NS3-4A serine protease. Antimicrob Agents Chemother 2008;52:110–20.
24. Tong X, Chase R, Skelton A, et al. Identification and analysis of fitness of resistance mutations against the HCV protease inhibitor SCH 503034. Antiviral Res 2006;70:28–38.
25. Schiff E, Poordad E, Jacobson I, et al. Boceprevir (B) combination therapy in null responders (NR): response dependent on interferon responsiveness [abstract]. J Hepatol 2008;48:S46.
26. Bartels DJ, Zhou Y, Zhang EZ, et al. Natural prevalence of hepatitis C virus variants with decreased sensitivity to NS3.4A protease inhibitors in treatment-naive subjects [see comment]. J Infect Dis 2008;198:800–7.
27. Kuntzen T, Timm J, Berical A, et al. Naturally occurring dominant resistance mutations to hepatitis C virus protease and polymerase inhibitors in treatment-naïve patients. Hepatology 2008;48:1769–78.
28. Howe AY, Ralston R, Chase R, et al. Favorable cross-resistance profile of two novel hepatitis C virus inhibitors, SCH-503034 and HCV-796, and enhanced anti-replicon activity mediated by the combined use of both compounds [abstract]. J Hepatol 2007;46:S165.
29. Flint M, Mullen S, Deatly AM, et al. Selection and characterization of hepatitis C virus replicons dually resistant to the polymerase and protease inhibitors HCV-796 and boceprevir (SCH 503034). Antimicrob Agents Chemother 2009; 53:401–11.

Telaprevir: Hope on the Horizon, Getting Closer

Ilan S. Weisberg, MD, MSc[a], Ira M. Jacobson, MD[b,*]

KEYWORDS

• Hepatitis C virus (HCV) • Protease inhibitor • Telaprevir
• STAT-C • NS3-4A

With more than 170 million people infected (roughly 3% of the world's population) hepatitis C virus (HCV) is a leading cause of chronic hepatitis, cirrhosis, and hepatocellular carcinoma,[1] and represents the commonest indication for liver transplantation in western nations. Current interferon-based treatment strategies are inadequate due to poor patient tolerability, prolonged treatment duration, and limited efficacy. For patients with genotype 1, the most prevalent form in the United States, standard treatment with 48 weeks of pegylated interferon and ribavirin achieves a sustained virologic response (SVR) rate of only about 40%.[2–5] This figure is even lower in African Americans and individuals with high viral load, advanced fibrosis, or HIV coinfection.[2,3,6–8] The availability of a well-tolerated, highly effective therapy for the treatment of chronic HCV remains a major unmet need.

Interferon is an indirectly acting antiviral agent that does not inhibit specific viral proteins or nucleic acids. The mechanism of action of ribavirin in HCV infection remains unclear. The search for direct antiviral agents that specifically target essential components of HCV replication has been the focus of intense research efforts. Using modern structure-based drug design techniques, small molecules that inhibit the HCV NS3-4A protease and the NS5B RNA-dependent RNA polymerase have emerged as the most promising of the specific targeted antiviral therapies for HCV (STAT-C). Telaprevir (VX-950, Vertex Pharmaceuticals), a peptidomimetic inhibitor of the NS3-4A protease in advanced stages of clinical development, shows great potential to favorably impact antiviral therapy for chronic HCV infection. In this review, the current experience with this new agent is summarized. Other HCV protease inhibitors, including boceprevir, another agent in phase 3 trials at the time of writing, are also under development and are covered elsewhere in this issue.

[a] Division of Gastroenterology and Hepatology, Department of Medicine, Center for the Study of Hepatitis C, Weill Cornell Medical College, 1305 York Ave, 4th Floor, New York Presbyterian Hospital, NY 10021, USA
[b] Division of Gastroenterology and Hepatology, Department of Medicine, Weill Cornell Medical College, 1305 York Ave, 4th Floor, New York Presbyterian Hospital, NY 10021, USA
* Corresponding author.
E-mail address: imj2001@med.cornell.edu (I.M. Jacobson).

Clin Liver Dis 13 (2009) 441–452
doi:10.1016/j.cld.2009.05.009
1089-3261/09/$ – see front matter

THE NS3-4A PROTEASE

The HCV RNA genome is translated as a single polyprotein precursor that is enzymatically processed by host and viral proteases.[9] The N-terminal portion of the polypeptide is processed by host cell proteases to generate 3 structural proteins (core, the E1 and E2 envelope glycoproteins) and p7 (an integral membrane protein whose function has not yet been definitively determined). The remainder of the polypeptide contains 6 nonstructural (NS) proteins required for viral replication and maturation, including NS3, a multifunctional enzyme with an N-terminal serine protease domain and a C-terminal RNA helicase/NTPase domain. With the addition of the NS4A cofactor essential for complete peptidase activity, the heterodimeric NS3-4A protease has substrate specificity distinct from that of host cell or other viral proteases.

Early in vitro and primate studies demonstrated the essential role of the NS3-4A protease and highlighted the therapeutic potential of an HCV protease inhibitor.[10,11] Chimpanzees inoculated with HCV clones with abrogated NS3-4A activity failed to generate productive HCV infection, suggesting that this protease is integral to viral replication and polypeptide maturation.[11] Furthermore, in vitro data have demonstrated that the NS3-4A protease may participate in host immune evasion by targeting for degradation several key cellular signaling molecules associated with endogenous interferon production and responsiveness.[12,13] The NS3-4A protease, therefore, may represent a dual therapeutic target by inhibiting viral replication and potentially restoring the innate response to chronic HCV infection.

These preclinical investigations paved the way for human trials with NS3-4A protease inhibitors. Proof of principle that HCV protease inhibition could efficiently and effectively suppress viral replication in vivo was established by the landmark study with ciluprevir (BILN2061) in genotype 1 treatment-naive or -experienced patients with chronic HCV infection.[14] With just 2 days of ciluprevir monotherapy, viral load reductions of 100- to 1000-fold were seen in all treated individuals. Although further progress with this molecule was halted due to concerns over cardiotoxicity in a monkey model,[15] the success with ciluprevir opened the door to future trials with NS3/4A protease inhibitors.

PRECLINICAL AND PHASE 1 TELAPREVIR DATA

Telaprevir is a selective peptidomimetic inhibitor of the HCV NS3-4A serine protease. It forms a covalent but reversible enzyme-inhibitor complex with a dissociation half-life of nearly 1 hour.[16] In vitro, telaprevir showed excellent antiviral activity in HCV replicon systems and purified human fetal hepatocytes exposed to sera infected with genotype 1a HCV.[16] Incubation of genotype 1b replicon cells with 2 weeks of telaprevir resulted in more than a 4-log reduction in HCV RNA level.[17] These in vitro data, coupled with a robust animal safety profile, allowed further development of telaprevir in human trials.

In an initial phase 1b dose-finding study,[18] 14 days of telaprevir monotherapy was well tolerated and demonstrated substantial antiviral activity. Thirty-four patients, 27 (79%) of whom had failed previous antiviral therapy, were treated with placebo or telaprevir at 450 mg every 8 hours, 750 mg every 8 hours, or 1250 mg every 12 hours. Decline in HCV RNA followed a biphasic pattern with an initial rapid decline followed by a second phase of gradual inhibition. The 750-mg group, which displayed the highest trough plasma drug concentrations, achieved a median reduction in HCV viral load of 4.4-log; the viral load became undetectable in 2 individuals after only 14 days of treatment. Viral rebound was seen in the 450-mg and 1250-mg groups and was attributed to the selection and proliferation of telaprevir-resistant variants.[18]

Having already established in replicon assays that interferon and telaprevir worked synergistically to inhibit HCV replication[19] and that telaprevir-resistant variants remained sensitive to interferon therapy,[20] a second phase 1 trial evaluating the combination of telaprevir and interferon a-2a was initiated.[21] Twenty treatment-naive subjects with genotype 1 chronic HCV infection were randomized to receive 2 weeks of pegylated interferon a-2a (180 μg weekly) with placebo, telaprevir monotherapy (1250 mg loading dose followed by 750 mg every 8 hours for 14 days), or interferon and telaprevir combination therapy. On completion of the study protocol, all participants were offered standard therapy for hepatitis C with pegylated interferon and ribavirin.

This study confirmed the antiviral effects of telaprevir and demonstrated that antiviral activity was enhanced when coadministered with interferon. Within 4 days of treatment, the combination of telaprevir 750 mg every 8 hours and pegylated interferon (peginterferon) a-2a 180 μg once weekly resulted in an initial rapid decline in HCV viral load followed by continued decline in HCV RNA throughout the 14-day dosing schedule.[21] At the end of the 2-week protocol, median reductions in HCV viral load of 1.0-, 4.0-, and 5.5-log were observed in individuals randomized to interferon, telaprevir, or the combination of the 2, respectively. After 12 weeks of standard HCV therapy with peginterferon and ribavirin, 5 of 7 (72%) patients initially treated with telaprevir and all 8 (100%) of the individuals treated with the telaprevir/interferon combination had undetectable HCV RNA. By week 24 of follow-on therapy, all 15 participants had undetectable virus, including those with documented resistance mutations, demonstrating the activity of standard therapy against the resistant variants. SVR data from this small study have been reported recently,[22] suggesting that telaprevir-based regimens may increase the chance of cure in genotype 1 chronic HCV infection. Of the 15 participants randomized to telaprevir or telaprevir/interferon before treatment with 24 or 48 weeks of standard HCV therapy, 9 (60%) achieved an SVR compared with only 1 of the 4 (25%) who was pretreated with interferon monotherapy.

One year later, results from the final phase 1 study, which evaluated using triple therapy with telaprevir, ribavirin, and interferon, were reported.[23] Using a single-arm, open-label study design, 12 treatment-naive genotype 1 subjects were given telaprevir (1250 mg loading dose followed by 750 mg 3 times daily), peginterferon a-2a (180 μg subcutaneous injection weekly), and weight-based ribavirin (1000–1200 mg daily) for a total of 28 days. Triple therapy was well tolerated and led to an unparalleled antiviral response; all 12 patients achieved a rapid virologic response (RVR) with undetectable virus by day 28. After the initial dosing period, all participants were offered 44 additional weeks of standard HCV therapy with peginterferon a-2a and ribavirin, and 8 ultimately went on to achieve an SVR. As seen in the previous combination study,[21] viral variants that emerged early in the dosing schedule continued to decline to levels of undetectability, supporting the evidence that these mutants remain susceptible to indirect antiviral agents such as interferon and ribavirin, thereby solidifying their role in future telaprevir study designs.

PHASE 2 TELAPREVIR DEVELOPMENT: THE PROVE TRIALS

Results from PROVE 1, the first North American multicenter telaprevir trial, demonstrated potent antiviral effects, low incidence of viral relapse, and the potential to shorten the total treatment duration for genotype 1 HCV infection.[24,25] In this large controlled study, 250 treatment-naive, genotype 1 HCV-infected individuals were randomized to receive telaprevir 750 mg every 8 hours, weekly injection with peginterferon a-2a 180 μg, and ribavirin 1000 to 1200 mg daily for 12 weeks followed by zero (n = 17), 12 (n = 79), or 36 (n = 79) additional weeks of peginterferon a-2a and ribavirin. Patients in the telaprevir arms with shorter treatment duration were eligible to stop treatment at those early time points only if HCV RNA was undetectable at week 4. A fourth control arm (n = 75) was given the standard of care for genotype 1 HCV, 48 weeks of pegylated interferon and weight-based ribavirin. Compared with controls, a significantly higher proportion of individuals in the 3 telaprevir-containing arms achieved undetectable HCV virus at weeks 4 (79% versus 11%, *P*<.001) and 12 (70% versus 39%, *P*<.001).

Unlike the 23% relapse rate observed in the control arm, only 2% of patients who had undetectable HCV RNA at weeks 4 and 12 on triple therapy had viral relapse after completing a course of 12 additional weeks of interferon and ribavirin. Furthermore, individuals in this 24-week course of treatment achieved SVR rates significantly higher than those in the 48-week control arm (61% versus 41%), demonstrating that the addition of telaprevir may allow for an abbreviated course of treatment with enhanced rates of virologic cure. SVR in the 48-week telaprevir-treated group was 67%, with a relapse rate of 6%. By contrast, only 35% of patients in the 12-week treated cohort had an SVR, with 3 of 9 (33%) of those having negative HCV RNA at week 4 and week 12 relapsing after discontinuing treatment. Although telaprevir was generally well tolerated, discontinuations due to adverse events such as rash, pruritus, anemia, and gastrointestinal disturbances were more frequent for the pooled telaprevir recipients versus controls during the initial 12 week dosing period (18% vs 4%) and overall (21% vs 11%). Severe rash represented the greatest incremental adverse event compared with control, with 7% of telaprevir-treated patients versus 1% of control patients discontinuing for this reason.

In the European counterpart study, PROVE 2, the combination of telaprevir, interferon, and ribavirin was similarly evaluated in genotype 1, treatment-naive HCV infection.[26,27] A total of 332 patients were randomized to 1 of 4 treatment groups including a 48-week control arm with telaprevir-matched placebo (PR48, n = 82), 12 weeks of telaprevir, interferon, and ribavirin triple therapy (T12/PR12, n = 82), a 24-week regimen consisting of 12 weeks of triple therapy followed by 12 additional weeks of interferon and ribavirin (T12/PR24, n = 81), and an ambitious ribavirin-sparing arm consisting of 12 weeks of peginterferon and telaprevir (T12/P12, n = 78). The size of the 12-week cohort was much larger in this study than in PROVE 1, and the latter had no ribavirin-free arm. Unlike PROVE 1, however, PROVE 2 had no 48-week telaprevir-based treatment arm.

As seen in PROVE 1, telaprevir was associated with potent antiviral activity and the potential to halve treatment duration while improving SVR rates significantly over routine care. Triple therapy with telaprevir, interferon, and ribavirin led to increased rates of RVR (74% versus 14%) and early virologic response (EVR) (79% versus 43%) over standard treatment.[27] The SVR rates in the 12 week (T12/PR12) and 24 week telaprevir arms (T12/PR24) were 60% and 69%, respectively, compared with only 46% of individuals in the control arm. The results of treatment in the ribavirin-free arm have far-reaching impact given the intense prevailing interest in the possibility of supplanting ribavirin with STAT-C agent. In this arm (T12/P12) only 51% and 62%, and 36% of individuals achieved an RVR, EVR, and SVR, respectively. Moreover, on-treatment virologic breakthrough (24% versus 1% in the T12/PR12 and 5% in the T12/PR24 arms) and off-treatment relapse (48%) were increased in the ribavirin-free arm. A major ramification of these data is the establishment of the importance of ribavirin in future HCV treatment. Again, telaprevir was well tolerated although dermatologic side effects (rash, pruritus) were more common and rashes more severe (6% with grade III) than in patients given standard therapy.[26]

PROVE 3 is an ongoing, randomized, placebo-controlled phase 2b trial being conducted at more than 50 centers in the United States, Canada, and Europe.[28] Four hundred and fifty-three patients who failed previous interferon-based treatment due to nonresponse, viral breakthrough, or relapse were randomized to 1 of 4 study arms including 12 weeks of triple therapy followed by 12 more weeks of interferon and ribavirin (T12/PR24), an extended telaprevir dosing arm consisting of 24 weeks of triple therapy followed by 24 additional weeks of interferon and ribavirin (T24/PR48), a 24-week ribavirin-sparing arm (T24/P24), and a standard therapy control arm (PR48). Patients randomized to the control arm who failed to achieve rapid or early virologic suppression were rolled over into a separate telaprevir-based protocol. Interim data from this important treatment failure study were recently reported.[28]

The most robust response was observed in the 24-week triple-therapy regimen (T12/PR24); the ribavirin-sparing arm (T24/P24) again showed weakened antiviral activity, and extending telaprevir dosing beyond 12 weeks (T24/P24 or T24/PR48) did not seem to offer any additional benefit. Of the 115 patients randomized to 24-week triple therapy (T12/PR24), 60 (52%) had undetectable virus 12 weeks post treatment (SVR-12). Although former relapsers had the best response to retreatment with a telaprevir-based regimen (29/40, 73%), SVR-12 also was notable in previous nonresponders (27/66, 41%) and individuals with viral breakthrough (4/9, 44%). The safety profile of PROVE 3 was similar to that of PROVE 1 and 2, with the most common reason for treatment discontinuation being rash (7%). Final SVR results are anticipated later this year.

These data represent a dramatic improvement over historical SVR rates (<20%) in patients with previous treatment failure.[29,30] One limitation of the PROVE 3 study was the unavailability of data allowing for stratification of patients by previous response pattern, for example, null versus partial response. This issue has been addressed in an ongoing "rollover" study in which patients who received standard of care therapy in the control arms of the 3 phase 2 telaprevir trials were offered re-treatment with open-label telaprevir combined with peginterferon and ribavirin for 12 weeks followed by 12 or 36 weeks of additional treatment with standard therapy. An interim analysis presented by Shiffman and colleagues[31] at AASLD 2008 showed that null responders, defined as patients with less than 1-log reduction in HCV RNA by week 4 or less than 2-log reduction by week 12 of prior therapy had HCV RNA clearance in 61% after 12 weeks of retreatment with triple therapy. However, response rates dropped to 43% at week 24. Genomic sequencing data to characterize the viral variants present at the time of the viral breakthroughs occurring after cessation of telaprevir are awaited, as are additional data on end of treatment response and sustained response. As expected, patients with prior partial response or relapse have higher rates of treatment response to telaprevir-based therapy. Whatever the rates of SVR ultimately prove to be, the study provides an intriguing proof of concept that even null responders to interferon and ribavirin can have a marked decline in viremia when a protease inhibitor is added to a retreatment regimen. This result raises a question as to whether HCV protease inhibition upregulates interferon-stimulated genes, as has been speculated in the face of evidence that the viral protease impedes innate immunity through well-documented pathways.[32]

Interim results from another trial have recently been reported[33] in which the therapeutic potential of twice daily telaprevir in combination with either of the 2 commercially available peginterferon preparations is being evaluated. This open-label trial involves 161 treatment-naive, genotype 1–infected HCV patients treated with 12 weeks of telaprevir at 750 mg every 8 hours or 1125 mg every 12 hours in combination with peginterferon a-2a (180 μg/wk) and ribavirin (1000–1200 mg daily), or peginterferon a-2b (1.5 μg/kg/wk) and ribavirin (800–1200 mg daily). Although there were no statistical differences noted, a trend toward higher RVR rates was noted in the 2 peginterferon a-2a arms (82% and 85% for TVR 750 mg PO every 8 hours and 1125 mg PO every 12 hours, respectively) compared with the 2 peginterferon a-2b arms (71% and 68% for TVR 750 mg PO every 8 hours and 1125 mg PO every 12 hours, respectively). Early virologic breakthrough seems equivalent in all groups. At this early stage, the true value of twice-a-day telaprevir and the impact of the type of peginterferon used remains unclear (note the difference in the ribavirin dosing range). The planned 12-week interim analysis and final SVR data will help clarify these outstanding issues.

PHASE III TELAPREVIR DEVELOPMENT: ADVANCE, ILLUMINATE, AND REALIZE

Several large, phase 3 telaprevir trials are now underway in treatment-naive individuals. As of January 2009, the ADVANCE trial (n = 1050) and the ILLUMINATE trial (n = 500) are fully enrolled with SVR data anticipated in 2010. The phase 3 program is cummulatively evaluating 24 or 48 weeks of telaprevir-based triple therapy versus 48 weeks of standard care in HCV genotype 1, treatment-naive individuals. In addition, the REALIZE trial has also completed enrollment (n = 650) and hopes to confirm the efficacy of telaprevir in genotype 1 individuals with prior treatment failure. Similar phase 3 trials in treatment-naive and treatment-failure individuals have recently been initiated in Japan.

TELAPREVIR RESISTANCE

With the tremendous potential of direct NS3/4A protease inhibition comes the need to focus on the issue of emerging drug resistance. HCV, like other RNA and retroviruses, possesses a low-fidelity RNA polymerase that lacks proofreading capacity. Given the high rate of HCV replication ($\sim 10^{12}$ new viral particles generated daily), it is estimated that the inherently error-prone polymerase will allow point mutations to arise at each position in the HCV genome every day.[34] These variants can preexist as minor viral populations, so-called "quasispecies," and can serve as a rapid source of drug resistance in patients treated with STAT-C therapies.

Mutations conferring resistance to telaprevir were initially identified and characterized in vitro using genotype 1b replicon assays.[20,35] Substitution of the Ala (alanine)[156] residue in the protease catalytic domain with a serine (A156S), valine (A156V), or threonine (A156T) was associated with high-level telaprevir resistance and dramatically diminished replicative fitness. Using a highly sensitive sequencing assay, the A156S variant as well as 3 additional mutations conferring lower-level resistance (V36A/M, T54A, and R155K/T) were identified in HCV genotype 1-infected patients treated with 14 days of telaprevir monotherapy.[36] In addition, double mutations conferring high-level resistance with increased replicative fitness have been identified at positions 36/155 or 36/156.[37] These telaprevir-resistant variants have all been shown to retain full wild-type sensitivity to treatment with interferon when studied in vitro[35,38,39] and continued clinical responsiveness to interferon and ribavirin in vivo.[37]

The appearance of 3 additional mutations in vivo that were not previously recognized in the replicon assays is believed to reflect the different genetic barrier to resistance between genotype 1a and genotype 1b infection.[36,37] For example, in genotype 1a only a single nucleotide substitution is necessary to replace the Arg (argenine)[155] residue with lysine (R155K) or threonine (R155T) whereas in the genotype 1b replicon system 2 nucleotide substitutions are required. Indeed, in the telaprevir monotherapy study the V36M and R155K/T variants were exclusively identified in genotype 1a infection[36] and of the individuals in PROVE 1 who demonstrated viral breakthrough with known telaprevir resistance mutations, most occurred in genotype 1a-infected patients.[24]

A report from France recently caused concern by describing a treatment-naive genotype 1a patient harboring a dominant telaprevir resistance mutation (R155K).[40] This case raises the troublesome possibility of primary protease inhibitor resistance and highlights that viral fitness in vivo is likely to differ from person to person, reflecting a balance between host and viral influences. How and why a highly resistant variant with diminished replicative fitness (in vitro) could emerge and predominate in the absence of selective pressure is entirely unexplained. The immunobiology of the host clearly is critical in determining the relative replicative fitness of individual HCV variants.

To further characterize the prevalence of dominant resistance mutations in the treatment-naive general population, 2 large studies evaluating more than 1000 individuals without prior telaprevir exposure, collectively, have recently been reported.[41,42] In the study by Bartels and colleagues[41] most subjects had wild-type virus (98%); however, a small percentage of subjects (all with genotype 1a HCV) were dominantly infected with V36M (0.9%), R155K (0.7%), V170A (0.2%), or R109K (0.2%) resistant variants. Similarly, in the report by Kuntzen and colleagues[42] dominant resistance mutations were common. Of the 362 genotype 1a subjects, 3 (0.8%), 6 (1.7%), 2 (0.6%), and 7(1.9%) were predominantly infected with the low-level resistant variants R155K, V36L, V36M, and T54S, respectively. In addition, 2 subjects (1.4%) with genotype 1b virus had baseline T54S as the dominant viral species. To date, there are no reports of primary dominant infection with the highly resistant A156 variant, consistent with its known deleterious effect on in vitro viral fitness. Although early data suggest impaired response to protease inhibitor therapy,[41] the clinical significance of telaprevir resistance variants at baseline and the future role of pretreatment drug resistance testing remain unclear and will require further study.

As the protease inhibitor story continues to unfold, it is increasingly apparent that combination therapies with interferon or other STAT-C inhibitors are mandatory to prevent the emergence of drug resistance and treatment failure. Because many of the known telaprevir resistance mutations show cross-resistance to other protease inhibitors currently in development, it is unlikely that coadministration of multiple agents from this class alone will offer a substantial treatment advantage. Rather, future therapies might include telaprevir as part of a combination of drugs with nonoverlapping resistance profiles targeting distinct HCV viral enzymes (eg, nucleoside and nonnucleoside NS5B HCV polymerase inhibitors, NS5A inhibitors, and so forth) and modifiers of host factors that result in viral suppression by way of a variety of pathways (eg, nitazoxinide, nonimmunosuppressive cyclosporine analogues, or therapeutic vaccines).

TELAPREVIR: SAFETY AND TOXICITY

At this time, safety data are available for many hundreds of patients treated with telaprevir in the phase 1 and 2 trials. Telaprevir is generally well tolerated with an overall safety profile similar to standard pegylated interferon and ribavirin. Short-term side effects including gastrointestinal disturbance, rash, pruritus, and anemia are the most common events leading to discontinuations in the telaprevir study arms, with discontinuation rates exceeding those in the control arms, and all have been reversible on drug withdrawal. The long-term virologic consequences of treatment failure after telaprevir exposure are less clear. In patients with the emergence of resistant variants, wild-type virus quickly returns after discontinuation of telaprevir and constitutes an increasing proportion of the viral population, but it has not yet been established that there is a distinct time point at which the baseline viral profile is fully restored. Thus, the impact prior telaprevir exposure will have on future HCV treatment with regimens containing telaprevir or other protease inhibitors with similar resistance profiles is uncertain. Unlike HIV or hepatitis B virus (HBV), there are no reservoirs of infection or archived genomes with HCV infection, and longer follow-up is needed to answer this important question.

FUTURE DIRECTIONS

With phase 3 telaprevir data anticipated in the near future, along with data on another protease inhibitor, boceprevir, the promise of a commercially available HCV protease inhibitor(s) for stable genotype 1 HCV infection seems poised to become reality. The early experience with the protease inhibitor class implies a potential to dramatically alter the treatment paradigm for the vast majority of people living with chronic HCV infection, with the added potential benefit of shortened treatment duration. However, several important HCV patient populations have, thus far, been minimally represented or excluded from telaprevir clinical trials.

The impact of telaprevir on African Americans and other minority populations is not yet fully established but likely to be favorable. These patients carry a substantial burden of disease yet demonstrate poor treatment response to standard HCV therapy. Subgroup analysis from the PROVE 1 study[43] suggests that telaprevir may help "level the playing field." Compared with Caucasians, in whom SVR increased from 46% to 62% the addition of telaprevir increased SVR from 11% to 44% and 33% to 65% in African Americans and Latino participants, respectively.[43,44] These findings of enhanced virologic suppression need to be confirmed in the larger phase 3 trials.

Patients living with HIV/HCV coinfection represent a second major group of patients underserved by current HCV therapy. At the present time there are no data on telaprevir in this difficult-to-treat population. However, pharmacokinetic studies of telaprevir dosed with antiretroviral agents are planned (www.clinicaltrials.gov) and discussions with the US Food and Drug Administration (FDA) and European authorities are underway to develop an HIV/HCV coinfection program.

The role of telaprevir in genotype non-1 infection has been less extensively characterized. Because patients with genotype 2 or 3 infection already achieve SVR rates of more than 80% with only 24 weeks of standard HCV therapy,[45] the additional benefit of a protease inhibitor is unclear. Furthermore, protease inhibitors exhibit genotype specificity. Early interim results from two phase 2 studies in treatment-naive HCV patients with genotype 2/3 and 4 have recently been reported. After 15 days of telaprevir-based triple therapy, patients with genotype 2 and 3 achieved a mean HCV RNA reduction of 5.3 and 4.7 log IU/ml, respectively compared to a 4.0 and 4.5 log IU/ml decline with pegylated interferon and ribavirin alone[46] while genotype 4 patients achieved a 3.5 and 2.0 log IU/ml reduction with triple therapy or standard of care.[47] These preliminary data suggest that telaprevir has substantial antiviral activity against genotype 2 and 4 infection, but limited efficacy in genotype 3 patients. Final SVR data are anticipated early next year.

Patients with advanced liver and kidney disease represent additional treatment challenges. Although the ribavirin-sparing arms of the PROVE 2 and PROVE 3 telaprevir trials showed diminished efficacy, for ribavirin intolerant patients with end-stage renal disease telaprevir may substantially increase the chance of cure. For individuals with cirrhosis, telaprevir may improve the odds of SVR and, when combined with other

STAT-C therapies, may ultimately obviate the need for interferon, thereby preventing the risk of treatment-related decompensation. Drug interaction with immunosuppressive therapy is needed to understand the applicability of telaprevir in the posttransplant setting to prevent and treat HCV recurrence.

SUMMARY

Telaprevir, a potent inhibitor of the HCV NS3/4A protease, shows great promise in early clinical trials to dramatically impact the treatment of chronic HCV infection. For patients with genotype 1 HCV, 24-week triple therapy with telaprevir, interferon, and ribavirin is associated with an increase in rates of SVR from 41%–48% to 61%–68% compared with a 48-week standard interferon and ribavirin regimen. Side effects of telaprevir include rash, pruritus, anemia, and gastrointestinal upset. Coadministration with interferon and ribavirin is essential to minimize virologic breakthrough and prevent relapse. With STAT-C "cocktails" comprising a combination of small molecule inhibitors a coveted ultimate goal, the quantum leap forward that would be represented by the addition of telaprevir and other protease inhibitors to the current armamentarium of HCV therapies increasingly seems to be within reach.

REFERENCES

1. Available at: www.who.int/mediacentre/factsheets/fs164/en/index.html. Accessed February 1, 2009.
2. McHutchison JG, Gordon S, Schiff E, et al. Interferon alfa-2b alone or in combination with ribavirin as initial treatment for chronic hepatitis C. N Engl J Med 1998; 339:1485–92.
3. Fried MW, Shiffman M, Reddy K, et al. PegInterferon alfa-2a plus ribavirin for chronic hepatitis C virus infection. N Engl J Med 2002;347:975–82.
4. Jacobson IM, Brown RS Jr, Freilich B, et al. Peginterferon alfa-2b and weight-based or flat-dose ribavirin in chronic hepatitis C patients: a randomized trial. Hepatology 2007;46:971–81.
5. Sulkowski E, Lawitz ML, Shiffman AJ, et al. Final results of the IDEAL (individualized dosing efficacy versus flatdosing to assess optimal pegylated interferon therapy) phase IIIB study. J Hepatol 2008;48:S370–1.
6. Conjeevaram HS, Fried MW, Jeffers LJ, et al. Peginteferon and ribavirin treatment in African American and Caucasian American patients with hepatitis C genotype 1. Gastroenterology 2006;131:470–7.
7. Torriani F, Rodriguez-Torres M, Rockstroh J, et al. Peginterferon alfa-2a plus ribavirin for chronic hepatitis C virus infection in HIV-infected patients. N Engl J Med 2004;351:438–50.
8. Jacobson IM, Brown RS Jr, McCone J, et al. Impact of weight-based ribavirin with peginterferon alfa-2b in African Americans with hepatitis C virus genoytpe 1. Hepatology 2007;46:982–90.
9. Lindenbach BD, Rice CM. Unravelling hepatitis C virus replication from genome to function. Nature 2005;436:933–8.
10. Bartenschlager R, Ahlborn-Lake L, Mous J, et al. Nonstructural protein 3 of the hepatitis C virus encodes a serine-type proteinase required for the cleavage of the NS3/4 and NS4/5 junctions. J Virol 1993;67:3835–44.
11. Kolykhalov AA, Mihalik K, Feinstone SM, et al. Hepatitis C virus encoded enzymatic activities and conserved elements in the 3' nontranslated region are essential for virus replication in vivo. J Hepatol 2000;74:2046–51.

12. Foy E, Li K, Wang C, et al. Regulation of interferon regulatory factor-3 by the hepatitis C virus serine protease. Science 2003;300:1145–8.
13. Li K, Foy E, Ferreon JC, et al. Immune evasion by hepatitis C virus NS3/4A mediated protease cleavage of the toll like receptor 3 adaptor protein TRIF. Proc Natl Acad Sci U S A 2005;102:2992–7.
14. Lamarre D, Anderson PC, Bailey M, et al. An NS3 protease inhibitor with antiviral effects in humans infected with hepatitis C virus. Nature 2003;426:186–9.
15. Hinrichsen H, Benhamou Y, Wedemeyer, et al. Short-term antiviral efficacy of BILN 2061, a hepatitis C virus serine protease inhibitor, in hepatitis genotype 1 patients. Gastroenterology 2004;127:1347–55.
16. Perni RB, Almquist SJ, Byrn RA, et al. Preclinical profile of VX-950, a potent, selective, and orally bioavailable inhibitor of hepatitis C virus NS3-4A serine protease. Antimicrob Agents Chemother 2006;50:899–909.
17. Lin K, Perni RB, Kwong AD, et al. VX-950, a novel hepatitis C virus (HCV) NS3-4A protease inhibitor, exhibits potent antiviral activities in HCV replicon cells. Antimicrob Agents Chemother 2006;50:1813–22.
18. Reesink HW, Zeuzem S, Weegink CJ, et al. Rapid decline of viral RNA in hepatitis C patients treated with VX-950: a phase 1b, placebo-controlled, randomized study. Gastroenterology 2006;131:997–1002.
19. Lin K, Kwong AD, Lin C. Combination of hepatitis C virus NS3-4A protease inhibitor and alpha interferon synergistically inhibits viral RNA replication and facilitates viral RNA clearance in replicon cells. Antimicrob Agents Chemother 2004;48:4784–92.
20. Lin C, Lin K, Luong YP, et al. In vitro resistance studies of hepatitis C virus serine protease inhibitors, VX-950 and BILN 2061. J Biol Chem 2004;279:17508–14.
21. Forestier N, Reesink HW, Weegink CJ, et al. Antiviral activity of Telaprevir (VX-950) and peginterferon alfa-2a in patients with hepatitis C. Hepatology 2007;46:640–8.
22. Weegink CJ, Forestier N, Jansen PL, et al. Final results of patients receiving Peg-Interferon-Alfa-2a (Ped-IFN) and ribavirin (RBV) after a 14-day study of the hepatitis C protease inhibitor telaprevir (VX-950) with Peg-IFN [abstract]. Hepatology 2007;S46:819A.
23. Lawitz E, Rodriguez-Torres M, Muir AJ, et al. Antiviral effects and safety of Telaprevir, peginterferon alfa-2a, and ribavirin for 28 days in hepatitis C patients. J Hepatol 2008;49:163–9.
24. Jacobson IM, Everson GT, Gordon SC, et al. Interim analysis results from a phase 2 study of telaprevir with peginterferon alfa-2a and ribavirin in treatment-naïve subjects with hepatitis C. Hepatology 2007;46:315A–6A.
25. McHutchison JG, Everson GT, Gordon SC, et al. Telaprevir with peginterferon and ribavirin for chronic HCV genotype 1 infection. N Engl J Med 2009;360:1827–38.
26. Hézode C, Forestier N, Dusheiko G, et al. Telaprevir and peginterferon with or without ribavirin for chronic HCV infection. N Engl J Med 2009;360:1839–50.
27. Zeuzem S, Hezode C, Ferenci P, et al. Telaprevir in combination with peginterferon alfa-2a with or without ribavirin in the treatment of chronic hepatitis C. Final Results of the PROVE 2 study. Hepatology 2008;48(S1):418A–9A.
28. McHutchison JG, Shiffman ML, Terrault N, et al. A Phase 2b study of telaprevir with peginterferon alfa-2a and ribavirin in hepatitis C genotype 1 null and partial responder and relapsers following a prior course of peginterferon alfa2a/b and ribavirin therapy. PROVE 3 interim results [abstract]. Hepatology 2008;48(S1):431A–2A.

29. Shiffman ML, Di Bisceglie AM, Lindsay KL, et al. Peginterferon alfa-2a and ribavirin in patients with chronic hepatitis C who have failed prior treatment. Gastroenterology 2004;126:1015–23.
30. Poynard T, Schiff E, Terf R, et al. Sustained viral response (SVR) is dependent on baseline characteristics in the retreatment of previous alfa interferon/ribavirin (I/R) nonresponders (NR): Final results from the EPIC3 program [abstract]. J Hepatol 2008;48:S369.
31. Shiffman ML, Berg T, Poordad F, et al. A study of Telaprevir combined with peginterfeon-alfa-2a and ribavirin in subjects with well-documented non-response or relapse after previous peginterferon-alfa-2a and ribavirin treatment: Interim analysis [abstract]. Hepatology 2008;48(S1):1135A–6A.
32. Lau DT, Fish PM, Sinha M, et al. Interferon regulatory factor-3 activation, hepatic interferon stimulated gene expression, and immune cell infiltration in hepatitis C virus patients. Hepatology 2008;47:799–809.
33. Forns X, Marecellin P, Goeser T, et al. Phase 2 study of Telaprevir administered Q8H or Q12H with peginterferon alfa-2a or alfa-2b and ribavirin in treatment naïve patients with genotype 1 hepatitis C: week 12 interim results [abstract]. Hepatology 2008;48(S1):1136A–7A.
34. Neuman AU, Lam NP, Dahari H, et al. Hepatitis C virus dynamics in vivo and the antiviral efficacy of interferon alpha therapy. Science 1998;282:103–7.
35. Lin C, Gates CA, Rao BG, et al. In vitro studies of cross-resistance mutations against two hepatitis C virus serine protease inhibitors, VX-950 and BILN 2061. J Biol Chem 2005;280:36784–91.
36. Sarrazin C, Kieffer TL, Bartels D, et al. Dynamic hepatitis C virus genotypic and phenotypic changes in patients treated with the protease inhibitor telaprevir. Gastroenterology 2007;132:1767–77.
37. Kieffer TL, Sarrazin C, Miller JS, et al. Telaprevir and pegylated interferon-alpha-2a inhibit wild-type and resistant genotype 1 hepatitis C virus replication in patients. Hepatology 2007;46:631–9.
38. Zhou Y, Muh U, Hanzelka BL, et al. Phenotypic and structural analyses of hepatitis C virus NS3 protease Arg-155 variants. J Biol Chem 2007;282:22619–28.
39. Zhou Y, Bartels DJ, Hanzelka BL, et al. Phenotypic characterization of resistant Val-36 variants in hepatitis C virus NS3-4A serine protease. Antimicrob Agents Chemother 2008;52:110–20.
40. Colson P, Brouk N, Lembo, et al. Natural presence of substitution R155K within hepatitis C virus NS3 protease from a treatment-naïve chronically infected patient. Hepatology 2008;47:766–7.
41. Bartels DJ, Zhou Y, Zhang E, et al. Natural prevalence of HCV resistance variants with decreased sensitivity to NS3-4A protease inhibitors in treatment naïve subjects. J Infect Dis 2008;198:800–7.
42. Kuntzen T, Timm J, Berical A, et al. Naturally occurring dominant resistance mutations to hepatitis C virus protease and polymerase inhibitors in treatment-naïve patients. Hepatology 2008;48:1769–78.
43. Muir AJ, Lawitz EJ, McHutchison JG, et al. Viral responses in African-Americans, Latinos, and Caucasians in the US phase 2 study (PROVE1) of telaprevir with peginterferon alfa-2a and ribavirin in treatment naïve genotype 1 infected subjects with hepatitis C [abstract]. Hepatology 2008;48(S1):1131A–2A.
44. Jacobson IM, Everson GT, Gordon SC, et al. Telaprevir with peginterferon alfa-2a and ribavirin in treatment-naïve patients with hepatitis C, including African-Americans and those with bridging fibrosis: Subgroup analysis from the phase 2

PROVE 1 trial. 13th Abstract P-113. International Symposium on Viral Hepatitis and Liver Disease, Washington, DC, USA, March 20-24, 2009.
45. Shiffman ML, Suter F, Bacon BR, et al. Peginterferon alfa-2a and ribavirin for 16 or 24 weeks in HCV genotype 2 or 3. N Engl J Med 2007;357:124–34.
46. Foster GR, Hezode C, Bronowicki JP, et al. Activity of telaprevir alone or in combination with peginterferon alpha-2A and ribavirin in treatment-naive genotype 2 and 3 hepatitis-C patients: interim results of study C209 [abstract]. Hepatology 2009;50:S22.
47. Benhamou Y, Moussali J, Ratziu, et al. Results of a proof of concept study (C210) of telaprevir monotherapy and in combination with peginterferon alpha-2A and ribavirin in treatment-naive genotype 4 HCV patients [abstract]. Hepatology 2009;50:S6.

HCV NS5B Polymerase Inhibitors

James R. Burton, Jr., MD*, Gregory T. Everson, MD

KEYWORDS

- Hepatitis C • Polymerase inhibitors • Antiviral therapy
- Clinical trials • Nucleoside analog • Non-nucleoside analog

Chronic hepatitis C virus (HCV) infection affects approximately 4 million persons and is the major indication for liver transplantation in the United States.[1] The current standard for treatment of HCV is pegylated interferon in combination with ribavirin. Despite significant advances in treatment, only approximately 50% of patients of treated patients clear HCV infection.[2,3] Response rates are even lower in African Americans, patients with cirrhosis, immunosuppressed patients, the elderly, and those coinfectioned with HIV.[4–8] Given these difficult to treat populations and that 50% or more of treated patients fail to achieve viral clearance with current therapy, development of new novel therapies is desperately needed.

Hepatitis C belongs to the Flaviviridae family. It is an enveloped virus containing a positive-sense, single-stranded RNA genome. This genome encodes for structural proteins that form the capsid and envelope and nonstructural (NS) proteins required for viral replications. Host and viral proteases release structural proteins involved in viral assembly and replication. The NS3/4A protease cleaves NS proteins releasing NS5B, the RNA-dependent RNA polymerase. Newly developed drugs, designated as specifically targeted antiviral therapy against hepatitis C (STAT-C), inhibit either the HCV protease or polymerase.

SPECIFICALLY TARGETED ANTIVIRAL THERAPY AGAINST HEPATITIS C

Challenges in the development of STAT-C drugs have included inability to grow HCV in culture and lack of a robust animal model. In the laboratory phase of drug development, activity of STAT-C drugs is assayed primarily by biochemical enzymatic assays and the cell-based HCV replicon system. Promising STAT-C drugs are then subjected to clinical trials to define safety and efficacy. Before release of new drugs for treatment, the US Food and Drug Administration (FDA) requires 3 phases of clinical investigation: phase I, phase II, and phase III. Phase I trials use single- and multiple-dose

Department of Medicine, Division of Gastroenterology and Hepatology, University of Colorado, Denver, 1635 Aurora Court, B154, 7th Floor Anschutz Outpatient Pavilion, Aurora, CO 80045, USA
* Corresponding author.
E-mail address: james.burton@ucdenver.edu (J.R. Burton).

Clin Liver Dis 13 (2009) 453–465
doi:10.1016/j.cld.2009.05.001
liver.theclinics.com

studies to define safety and tolerability. Phase II trials are generally dose-finding, and phase III trials compare the new treatment with the existing standard of care, to define clinical usefulness, and potentially gain approval from the FDA.

A key goal in the development of STAT-C drugs is limiting emergence of viral resistance to the administered compounds. Viral resistance is detected clinically by rebound in HCV RNA after initial suppression and viral variants are defined by sequence analysis. The 2 main factors that increase risk for emergence of resistant variants are the potency of the STAT-C drug and use of monotherapy versus multidrug treatment regimens. STAT-C drugs with low potency are associated with limited reduction in HCV RNA levels and maintenance of higher levels of viral replication. The latter factors favor mutational events, which allow escape from suppression by the STAT-C drug. Multidrug regimens inhibit viral replication at more than 1 locus of replication; variants resistant to 1 drug in a multidrug regimen are often sensitive to 1 or several of the other drugs in the regimen. The best strategy to prevent viral resistance is use of multiple drugs, each with a high potency against HCV.

NUCLEOSIDE ANALOG VERSUS NON-NUCLEOSIDE POLYMERASE INHIBITORS

Viral polymerase inhibitors are currently the largest class of antiviral drugs for the treatment of hepatitis B, HIV, and herpes viruses, and were some of the first drugs developed for the treatment of HCV. A large proportion of these drugs are nucleoside analogs, synthetic compounds structurally similar to nucleosides, the building blocks of RNA and DNA. The NS5B polymerase inhibitors for treatment of chronic hepatitis C consist of 2 classes: (1) nucleoside or nucleotide inhibitors (active site inhibitors) and (2) non-nucleotide inhibitors (allosteric inhibitors).

Nucleoside inhibitors are analogs of natural substrates of the polymerase that are incorporated into the growing RNA chain leading to chain termination by binding the active site of NS5B. They must be phosphorylated before being active. Because NS5B is a highly conserved region of the HCV genome, nucleoside inhibitors have similar activity against all genotypes and high genetic barriers to resistance.[9]

In contrast to nucleoside inhibitors, non-nucleoside inhibitors achieve NS5B inhibition by binding to 1 of the at least 5 allosteric enzyme sites resulting in conformational changes of the protein-inhibiting catalytic activity of polymerase. They have genotype-specific activity and potential for rapid selection of resistance. The rapid development of resistant mutants is possible with non-nucleoside inhibitors because they bind distantly to the active center of NS5B and mutations at the non-nucleoside inhibitor binding site may not necessarily lead to impairment of the enzyme function. Due to their distinctive binding sites, different polymerase inhibitors could theoretically be used in combination to avoid development of resistance.[9]

Multiple factors affect antiviral potency of these drugs influencing their ability to achieve sustained virologic response.[10] In vivo factors include inherent potency of the drug, and pharmacokinetic and pharmacodynamic properties, such as C_{trough} levels, dosing frequency, tolerability, rate of absorption, tissue distribution, metabolism and elimination, and induction of cellular transport mechanisms. In addition, impaired intestinal absorption of nucleoside analogs requires formulation of prodrugs to improve their bioavailability.

Several HCV NS5B polymerase inhibitors have demonstrated clinical efficacy and advanced to clinical trials (**Table 1**). Currently only R1728 (Pharmasset/Roche) remains under active clinical investigation. **Table 2** summarizes the clinical trials to date using pegylated interferon and ribavirin in combination with polymerase inhibitors.

Table 1
HCV NS5B polymerase inhibitors under clinical investigation

Drug Name	Company	Study Phase
Nucleoside analog NS5B polymerase inhibitors		
Valopicitabine (NM283)/NM107[a]	Idenix/Novartis	Withdrawn
R1626/R1479[a]	Roche	Withdrawn
R7128/PS-6130[a]	Pharmasset/Roche	Phase II
IDX184	Idenix	Phase I
MK-0608	Merck	Preclinical
Non-nucleoside NS5B polymerase inhibitors		
HCV-796	ViroPharma/Wyeth	Withdrawn
BILB 1941	Boehringer Ingelheim	Withdrawn
PF-868554	Pfizer	Phase II
GS 9190	Gilead	Phase II
VCH-759	ViroChem Pharma	Phase II
VCH-916	ViroChem Pharma	Phase I
GSK625433	GlaxoSmithKline	Phase I
ANA598	Anadys Pharmaceuticals	Phase I
ABT-333	Abbott	Phase I

[a] Prodrug/nucleoside analog.

NUCLEOSIDE ANALOG NS5B POLYMERASE INHIBITORS

Valopicitabine

Valopicitabine (NM203) is the oral prodrug of the nucleoside analog 2′-C-methyl-cytidine. The maximum effective dose was not defined because dosing was limited by the development of gastrointestinal side effects.

Clinical trials

The efficacy and safety of valopicitabine alone and in combination with pegylated interferon have been assessed in phase I and II clinical trials.[11–13] Studies of valopicitabine monotherapy indicated that a dose of 400 to 800 mg was optimal; higher doses were not well tolerated due to significant side effects, specially nausea and vomiting. Doses of 200 mg of valopicitabine were well tolerated in combination with peginterferon and effective. Studies in combination with ribavirin were not done due to increased gastrointestinal side effects.

One major phase IIb trial examining the combination of valopicitabine with peginterferon failed to demonstrate improved efficacy over the standard of care (SOC) of peginterferon/ribavirin.[13] Side effects requiring dose reductions in the higher dose peginterferon/valopicitabine arms limited efficacy and tolerability of this regimen. On review of the clinical data, the FDA revised the clinical trial of treating naive patients by reducing the dose of valopicitabine from 800 mg to 200 or 400 mg/d. Subsequent analysis by the FDA of the risk-benefit profile from the phase II clinical trial resulted in suspension of clinical development of valopicitabine in the United States.[14]

Prospects for future drug development

Although development of valopicitabine for the treatment of chronic hepatitis C in the United States has ceased, trials in Europe in combination with peginterferon/ribavirin

Table 2
Clinical trials of NS5B polymerase inhibitors in combination with peginterferon and ribavirin in HCV genotype 1

Drug (Company)	Reference	Antiviral History	Regimen	Mean Day 14 Decrease in HCV RNA (log_{10} IU/mL)	% HCV RNA Undetectable	
					RVR	ETR
Nucleoside analogue inhibitors						
R7128/PS1-6130 (Pharmasset/Roche)	20	TF	1500 mg twice a day × 28 days	2.7	–	–
	40	TN	1500 mg twice a day with peg/riba (versus SOC) × 28 days	5.1 (3.0) at 28 days	85	–
R1626/R1479 (Roche)	15	TN	1500 mg twice a day × 14 days	1.2	–	–
	16	TN	1500 mg twice a day with peg/riba (versus SOC) × 48 days	4.6 (1.6)	74 (5)	84 (65)
Non-nucleoside inhibitors						
HCV-796 (Virochem/Wyeth)	41	TN	1000 mg twice a day × 14 days	0.8 increase	–	–
	29	TN	1000 mg twice a day with peg × 14 days (versus peg alone)	Range 2.6–3.2 (1.2)	–	–

Abbreviations: ETR, End-of-treatment response, HCV RNA undetectable at week 12; RVR, Rapid virological response, HCV RNA undetectable at week 4; SOC, Standard of care (pegylated interferon [peg] and ribavirin [riba]); TF, Treatment failure; TN, Treatment naive.

are ongoing. Results of these latter trials will determine the ultimate fate of valopicitabine.

R1626

R1626 is a tri-isobutyl ester prodrug of the nucleoside analog R1479 (4′-azidocytidine). It is rapidly converted by esterases in gastrointestinal epithelial cells to R1479, whereby it is phosphorylated and becomes a potent and highly selective terminator of HCV NS5B.

Clinical trials

Two studies were published in *Hepatology* (summarized later) at or about the same time Roche announced that development of R1626 was terminated due to "new and unexpected safety findings" from the phase IIb study (POLI 1) (Roche earning report, October 21, 2008).

Roberts and colleagues published results of an observer-blinded, randomized, placebo-controlled, multiple ascending dose phase Ib study in 47 genotype-1 patients naive to treatment.[15] Patients were randomized to receive R1626 orally at doses of 500 mg, 1500 mg, 3000 mg or 4500 mg or matched placebo twice daily for 14 days. After oral administration, R1626 was efficiently converted to R1479 with near dose proportional pharmokinetics (57%–71% R1626 converted to R1479 over 12 hours after the last dose of R1626 on day 14). Mean decreases in HCV RNA blood levels were 0.32, 1.2, 2.6, and 3.7 $\log_{10}$ for the respective treatment arms.

R1626 was generally well tolerated up to 3000 mg twice a day with only mild side effects in 67% of cases. Gastrointestinal symptoms (diarrhea and nausea) were common, especially in the group taking 4500 mg twice a day. In addition, there was pancytopenia suggesting bone marrow suppression with a dose of 4500 mg twice a day. For these reasons, future clinical trials were limited to 3000 mg twice a day or less.

Three patients exhibited viral rebound (viral load reduction 0.5 $\log_{10}$ IU/mL or greater followed by a 0.5 $\log_{10}$ or greater increase in HCV RNA level from nadir during treatment). These 3 patients all received a dose of 500 mg twice a day. Pre- and end-of-treatment samples from these 3 patients showed no common amino acid changes and no significant changes in susceptibility to R1479 attributed to inadequate drug levels. Three additional patients from the group on a dose of 500 mg showed no response to drug throughout treatment. Again, nonresponse was attributed to inadequate drug. There was no evidence of viral resistance from phenotypic and sequencing analysis to known 1479-resistant NS5B mutations (S96T or S96T/N142T). In contrast to other observations to date with other antivirals, no selection of resistance to R1479 despite inadequate drug levels was seen.

Pockros and colleagues examined the safety and efficacy of dosing R1626 for 28 days in combination with peginterferon or peginterferon/ribavirin.[16] There were 4 treatment arms in this trial: DUAL 1500 (1500 mg twice a day R1626 + peginterferon), DUAL 3000 (3000 mg twice a day R1626 + peginterferon), TRIPLE 1500 (1500 mg twice a day R1626 + peginterferon + ribavirin), and SOC (peginterferon + ribavirin).

The study randomized 107 patients to receive 28 days of R1626 (1500 mg or 3000 mg twice daily) with either peginterferon (DUAL arms) or peginterferon/ribavirin (TRIPLE arm). After day 28, all patients were treated for an additional 44 weeks with peginterferon/ribavirin to complete a 48-week course of treatment. Results were compared with SOC. Growth factors were discouraged initially; however the study was amended such that investigators were advised to manage treatment-related adverse events according to their "best clinical judgment," which may have included growth factors (erythropoietin or granulocyte-colony stimulating factor).

The study was double blinded until all patients received 8 weeks of treatment (4 weeks of R1626 or placebo, plus the first 4 weeks of SOC). Baseline patient demographics were equally matched with most patients being Caucasian (89%), male (64%), and genotype 1a (77%). Mean baseline HCV RNA levels were similar (6.5–6.7 $\log_{10}$ IU/mL). A strong antiviral effect for R1626 with peginterferon with and without ribavirin was observed; the mean reduction in HCV RNA was 2.4, 3.6, 4.5, and 5.2 $\log_{10}$ for SOC, DUAL 1500, DUAL 3000, and TRIPLE 1500 arms, respectively.

Combining the results from the Roberts and Pockros studies suggests that peginterferon is synergistic with and not simply additive to R1626 in the suppression of HCV RNA. In the monotherapy trial of Roberts, the dose of 1500 mg twice a day was associated with a mean decrease of 1.2 $\log_{10}$, or median of 0.8 $\log_{10}$ in HCV RNA. Peginterferon monotherapy would be associated with $\sim$0.5 $\log_{10}$ decrease in HCV RNA. If peginterferon were simply additive to R1626 then the maximum decrease in HCV RNA with the combination of peginterferon + R1626 would be less than 2.0 $\log_{10}$. In fact, a median decrease of 3.1 $\log_{10}$ in HCV RNA was observed, consistent with synergism. The investigators also propose a similar synergism with the addition of ribavirin, already previously described in vivo.[17] The molecular mechanism for this antiviral synergy is not known.

Most adverse events were mild (80%) or moderate (16%). Most side effects were attributed to peginterferon (nausea, headache, and fatigue). As in the monotherapy study, gastrointestinal side effects were most commonly seen in the 3000 mg twice a day arm (diarrhea, 75%; nausea, 69%). Patients receiving R1626 were more likely to have hematological changes (neutropenia and anemia). Grade IV neutropenia occurred in 53% of patients in the 3000 mg arm with 25% receiving filgrastim. This degree of neutropenia was not seen in the monotherapy study suggesting that this observation was a consequence of combining R1626 with peginterferon. The largest decrease in hemoglobin at 4 weeks was observed in the arm receiving R1626 and ribavirin (32% with Hb <10 g/dL versus 5% in the SOC arm). The investigators state there was no evidence of hemolysis, therefore they postulate that it may be associated with reversible decreased red blood cells from bone marrow.

Resistance to R1429 was assessed in patients with viral rebound ($\geq$0.5 $\log_{10}$ IU/mL decrease in HCV RNA followed by a subsequent on-treatment increase of $\geq$0.5 $\log_{10}$ IU/mL above nadir). Eight patients had viral rebound during the 4-week treatment period, however all 8 had discontinued R1626 because of neutropenia before experiencing viral rebound. Samples from these patients revealed no change in susceptibility to R1470. Sequence analysis of the entire NS5B coding region revealed no known R1479 resistance mutations (S96T or S96T/N142T) or any other amino acid substitutions compared with the baseline sequence.

In mid-2008, end-of-treatment response (ETR; undetectable HCV RNA at 48 weeks of therapy) results were presented from the phase IIa study.[18] Eighty-four percent of patients receiving R1626 1500 mg twice a day with SOC achieve ETR compared with 65% group D receiving SOC. **Fig. 1** summarizes virological response rates during and 24 weeks after the end of the study (equivalent to sustained virological response, SVR).[19] The high rate of relapse is likely due to the short period of R1626 dosing (4 weeks).

Prospects for future drug development

R1626 has been withdrawn from further consideration for future drug development in the treatment of chronic hepatitis C. Two major factors led to this decision by the

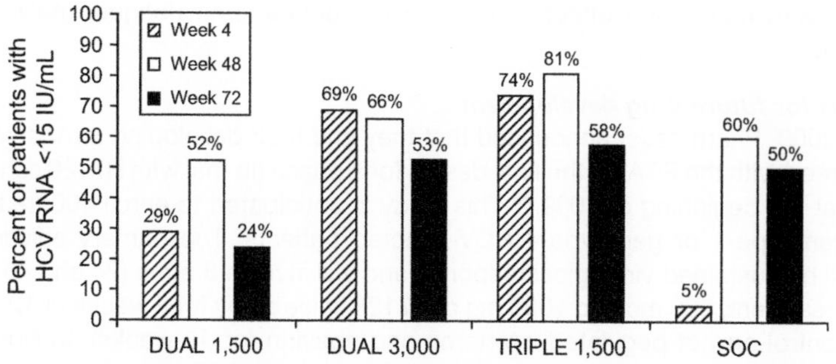

Fig. 1. Virological response rates during and 24 weeks after the end of treatment (72 weeks) in a phase IIa study with R1626 and pegylated interferon ± ribavirin.[22] DUAL 1,500, 1500 mg R1626 twice a day + 180 μg peginterferon alfa-2a weekly × 4 weeks, then SOC × 44 weeks; DUAL 3,000, 3000 mg R1626 twice a day + 180 μg peginterferon alfa-2a weekly × 4 weeks, then SOC × 44 weeks; TRIPLE 1,5000, 1500 mg R1626 + 180 μg peginterferon alfa-2a weekly + 1000 to 1200 mg ribavirin daily × 4 weeks, then SOC; SOC, standard of care (peginterferon alfa-2a weekly + 1000 to 1200 mg ribavirin daily) × 48 weeks.

manufacturer: suspicion for significant bone marrow suppression with even short courses of treatment and lack of superior efficacy with the studied regimens, compared with SOC.

R7128

R7128, a prodrug of PSI-6130, is an oral cytidine nucleoside analog polymerase inhibitor. In dose-response studies, there was an increase in virologic response with increasing dose, over a dose range from 750 mg daily every day to 1500 mg twice daily.

Clinical trials

A phase Ib clinical study demonstrated a mean HCV RNA reduction of 2.7 $\log_{10}$ IU/mL when administered as monotherapy at 1500 mg twice a day for 2 weeks in treatment-experienced patients infected with genotype 1.[20] In this study no serious adverse events were reported with more adverse events occurring in the placebo group.

In a phase IIa study, 81 naive-to-therapy, genotype-1 patients were randomized across 3 cohorts (cohort 1, R7128 500 mg twice a day + peginterferon + ribavirin (SOC); cohort 2, R7128 1000 mg twice a day + SOC; and cohort 3, R7128 1500 mg twice a day + SOC; 20–25 active/5–6 placebo stratification) and treated for 28 days.[21] Baseline characteristics were similar in each group. Subjects receiving 1000 mg or 1500 mg twice a day + SOC achieved a rapid virologic response (HCV RNA <15 IU/mL at week 4) in 88% and 85%, respectively versus 19% for placebo + SOC. No apparent differences in HCV RNA reduction across race/ethnicity with respect to R7218 1000 or 1500 mg twice a day dosing. No dose-related changes in terms of safety and tolerability were noted. No serious adverse events were noted and most side effects were mild.

Preliminary data (up to day 56 in all) are available in 25 HCV genotype-2 and -3 patients (10 nonresponders, 15 relapsers to SOC) receiving R7128 1500 mg twice a day + SOC (n = 20) compared with placebo + SOC (n = 5) for 28 days.[22] Plasma HCV RNA levels decreased a mean of 5.0 $\log_{10}$ IU/mL (90% rapid virological response [RVR]) in the treatment group compared with 4.3 $\log_{10}$ IU/mL (60% RVR) in the placebo group. Again, no serious adverse events or dose-related side effects were reported with many side effects attributed to peginterferon (fatigue, malaise, and headache).

Prospects for future drug development

In early 2009, Pharmasset announced that they and their developing partner, Roche, have agreed with the FDA on the final design for a phase IIb trial with R7128 scheduled to start at the beginning of 2009.[23] This study is anticipated to enroll 400 treatment-naive, genotype-1 or genotype-4 HCV-infected patients. The primary efficacy end point will be sustained virological response and will involve 5 arms (24 and 48 weeks of total treatment, 500 mg and 1000 mg of R7128 twice a day for 8 weeks or 12 weeks, and a control arm of pegylated interferon and ribavirin for 48 weeks). In November 2008, Pharmasset, Roche, and InterMune initiated the INFORM-1 trial to investigate the combination of R7128 with InterMune's protease inhibitor (ITMN-191).

IDX184

In January 2009, Idenix announced that it will study its polymerase inhibitor, IDX184, in HCV genotype-1 treatment-naive patients who will receive 1 of 4 doses (25 to 100 mg once a day). The study will include 10 patients who will receive the study drug and 2 patients who will receive a placebo drug. Unlike first-generation HCV nucleoside inhibitors (valopicitabine, R7128, and R1626), IDX184 is a "liver-targeted" prodrug, which theoretically will provide increased anti-HCV efficacy and safety. Preliminary studies in monkeys have shown ~95% hepatic extraction of orally administered IDX184 with low systemic IDX184 and nucleoside metabolite levels.[24] In chimpanzees infected with HCV genotype 1, once daily oral administration of 10 mg/kg/d of IDX184 produced mean viral load reduction of 2.3 $\log_{10}$ after 4 days of dosing.[25]

MK-0608

MK-0608 (Merck) is a potent nucleoside analog in preclinical trials.[26]

NON-NUCLEOSIDE NSB5 POLYMERASE INHIBITORS

HCV-796

HCV-796 is a benzofuran-C3-carboxamide non-nucleoside inhibitor of the HCV NS5B polymerase. In vitro studies using the replicon system showed that multiple treatments with HCV-796 resulted in 3 to 4 $\log_{10}$ reduction in HCV RNA levels, compared with 2 to 3 $\log_{10}$ reduction with interferon.[27]

Clinical trials

Preliminary phase I studies reported favorable results for HCV-796 administered as a single dose in health volunteers.[28] Phase Ib studies for up to 14 days in genotype-1 patients revealed a mean reduction in HCV RNA from baseline at day 7 and day 14 ranging from 1.5 to 2.3 $\log_{10}$ (versus mean 0.9 $\log_{10}$ for peginterferon alone) and 2.6 to 3.2 $\log_{10}$ (versus mean 1.3 $\log_{10}$ for peginterferon alone), respectively.[29,30] In combination with peginterferon, HCV-796 reduced HCV RNA up to 3.2 $\log_{10}$ at day 14 compared with 1.7 $\log_{10}$ with peginterferon alone.[29] In these studies HCV-796 exhibited favorable tolerability and no dose-limiting toxicity up to 14 days. A study of HCV-796 with peginterferon and ribavirin in a phase II study was suspended due to safety concerns after elevated liver enzymes were identified in 8% of patients, compared with 1% of controls.[31] The week 4 and week 12 results of this study were presented at the European Study of Liver Disease Annual Meeting in 2009 and demonstrated that HCV-796 had effective antiviral activity and improved RVR and early virological response (EVR) in genotype-1 subjects when used in combination with PEG-Intron and ribavirin (RBV).[32]

Prospects for future drug development

There are no ongoing trials of HCV-796. The drug has been removed from further consideration by Wyeth, the manufacturer. Although this compound will not be further developed due to unexpected elevations in liver enzymes, other non-nucleoside polymerase inhibitors are in development and may be effective in genotype-1 HCV.

BILB 1941

BILB 1941 (Boehringer Ingelheim) is non-nucleoside polymerase inhibitor. In a phase I trial, BILB 1941 had potent antiviral activity at 5 days in 96 HCV genotype-1 patients.[33] Gastrointestinal intolerance at higher doses, elevated liver enzymes, and its liquid formulation led to a halt in further development.

PF-00868554

PF-00868554 (Pfizer) is a non-nucleoside polymerase inhibitor under development by Pfizer. In an 8-day, phase I study, 32 treatment-naive genotype-1 HCV patients received PF-00868554 at different doses (100, 300, or 450 mg twice daily, or 300 mg 3 times daily) with mean reduction in HCV RNA at day 8 of 0.68, 1.26, 1.21, and 1.95 $\log_{10}$, respectively.[34] A study of PF-00868554 in combination with peginterferon and ribavirin in treatment-naive patients is currently underway.

GS 9190

GS 9190 (Gilead) is another non-nucleoside polymerase inhibitor under development. It has exhibited potent antiviral activity in the replicon system (higher activity in genotype-1 replicons compared with genotype-2).[35] A phase I study included 31 treatment-naive genotype-1 patients receiving a single dose of GS 9190 (40–480 mg).[36] The drug was well tolerated and pharmacokinetics of the drug support once daily or twice daily dosing. Median HCV RNA reduction at 24 hours ranged from ~0.7 to 1.2 $\log_{10}$ IU/mL across all cohorts. Preliminary data of 23 study participants who received multiple ascending doses over 8 days suggested that GS 9190 may be associated with QT prolongation. After expert consultation and a separate dose-ranging study in healthy volunteers, Gilead felt that the QT prolongation at a lower dose of the drug was "clinically manageable" (Gilead Quarterly Report, May 2, 2008). Gilead has begun recruitment for a phase II study of GS 9190 in combination with peginterferon and ribavirin for a treatment duration of 24 or 48 weeks.

VCH-759

VCH-759 (ViroChem Pharma) is a non-nucleoside polymerase inhibitor under investigation. In a 10-day, phase I study in 32 treatment-naive genotype-1 HCV patients receiving VCH-759 at different doses (400 mg 3 times daily, 800 mg twice daily and 800 mg 3 times daily), all achieved at least a 1 $\log_{10}$ drop in HCV RNA with the higher dosing regimen achieving a 2.5 $\log_{10}$ drop.[37] Phase II trials of VCH-759 are currently underway.

VCH-916

VCH-916 (ViroChem Pharma) is a non-nucleoside polymerase inhibitor. Preclinical and phase I trials of healthy volunteers at single doses of 50 to 600 mg have found it to be generally safe, highly absorbed, and well tolerated.[38] Studies in HCV patients are currently recruiting patients.

GSK625433

GSK625433 (GlaxoSmithKline) is a non-nucleoside polymerase inhibitor that is currently under phase I study.

ANA598

ANA598 (Anadys Pharmaceuticals) is a non-nucleoside polymerase inhibitor under investigation. In January 2009, Anadys announced the results from a study of 10 patients (8 received ANA598, 2 received placebo). The 8 patients who completed 3 days of 200 mg of ANA598 twice daily experienced a median 2.5 (range 1.4–3.4) $\log_{10}$ decrease in HCV RNA.[39] The drug was safe and well tolerated. The second part of the study is currently enrolling.

ABT-333

In June 2008, Abbott initiated a phase I, double-blind, randomized, placebo-controlled trial in healthy and HCV genotype-1 patients to evaluate safety, tolerability, antiviral activity, and pharmacokinetics of their polymerase inhibitor, ABT-333. The study is concluded in February 2009.

SUMMARY

The emergence of STAT-C drugs makes this an exciting time for patients with chronic HCV infection and those who care for them. Polymerase inhibitors, given their potent antiviral effects, represent a major contribution to the future of HCV treatment. Despite the enthusiasm these drugs have created, numerous questions regarding safety, tolerability, efficacy, and resistance profiles remain to be answered by ongoing and future clinical trials. The low genetic barrier for non-nucleoside inhibitors will likely require their combination with protease inhibitors and other polymerase inhibitors, as well as pegylated interferon and ribavirin. Whether these new drugs will have a role in the treatment of the difficult patient (nonresponders, those coinfected with HIV, decompensated liver disease and liver transplant recipients) remains to be determined.

REFERENCES

1. National Institutes of Health Consensus Development Conference Statement: Management of hepatitis C: 2002–June 10–12, 2002. Hepatology 2002;36(5 Suppl 1):S3–20.
2. Mann MP, McHutchison JG, Cordon SC, et al. Peginterferon alfa-2b plus ribavirin compared with interferon alfa-2b plus ribavirin for initial treatment of chronic hepatitis C: a randomized trial. Lancet 2001;358:958–65.
3. Fried MW, Shiffman ML, Reddy KR, et al. Peginterferon alfa-2a plus ribavirin for chronic hepatitis C virus infection. N Engl J Med 2002;347:975–82.
4. Torriani FJ, Rodriguez-Torres M, et al. Peginterferon alfa-2a plus ribavirin for chronic hepatitis C virus infection in HIV-infected patients. N Engl J Med 2004; 351:438–50.
5. Chung TR, Andersen J, Volberding P, et al. Peginterferon alfa-2a plus ribavirin versus interferon alfa 2a plus ribavirin for chronic hepatitis C in HIV-coinfected persons. N Engl J Med 2004;351:451–9.
6. Conjeevaram HS, Fried MW, Jeffers LJ, et al. Peginterferon and ribavirin treatment in African American and Caucasian American patients with hepatitis C genotype 1. Gastroenterology 2006;131(2):470–7.

7. Mindikoglu AL, Miller RR. Hepatitis C in the elderly; epidemiology, natural history and treatment. Clin Gastroenterol Hepatol 2009;7:128–34.
8. Everson GT. Treatment of chronic hepatitis C in patients with decompensated cirrhosis. Rev Gastroenterol Disord 2004;4(Suppl 1):S31–8.
9. Mann MP, Foster GR, Rockstroh JK, et al. The way forward in HCV treatment – finding the right path. Nat Rev Drug Discov 2007;6:991–1000.
10. Kwong AD, McNair Lindsay, Jacobson I, et al. Recent progress in the development of selected hepatitis C virus NS3-4A protease and NS5B polymerase inhibitors. Curr Opin Pharmacol 2008;8:522–31.
11. Zhou XJ, Afdhal N, Godofsky E, et al. Pharmacokinetics and pharmacodynamics of valopicitabine (NM283), a new nucleoside HCV polymerase inhibitor: results from a phase I/II dose-escalation trial in patients with HCV-1 infection [abstract]. J Hepatol 2005;42:229A.
12. Godofsky EW, Afdal N, Rustgi V, et al. First clinical results for a novel antiviral treatment for hepatitis C: a phase I/III dose escalation trial assessing tolerance, pharmacokinetics and antiviral activity on NM283, a novel antiviral treatment for hepatitis C [abstract]. Gastroenterology 2004;126(Suppl 2):A681.
13. Afdhal N, O'Brian C, Godofsky E, et al. Valopicitabine (NM283), alone or with peginterferon, compared to peginterferon/ribavirin (PEGIFN/RBV) retreatment in patients with HCV-1 infection and prior non-response to PEGIFN/RBV: one-year results [abstract]. J Hepatol 2007;46:S5.
14. Valopicitabine development program placed on clinical hold in the United States [press release]. Cambridge (MA): Idenix Pharmaceuticals Inc; 2007.
15. Roberts SK, Cooksley G, Dore GJ, et al. Robust antiviral activity of R1626, a novel nucleoside analog: a randomized, placebo-controlled study in patients with chronic hepatitis C. Hepatology 2008;48:398–406.
16. Pockros PJ, Nelson D, Godofsky E, et al. R1626 plus peginterferon alfa-2a provides potent suppression of hepatitis C virus RNA and significant antiviral synergy in combination with ribavirin. Hepatology 2008;48:285–97.
17. Jiang W-R, Chiu S, Ali S, et al. In vitro antiviral interactions of a novel HCV inhibitor R1479 with interferon α2a, ribavirin and other HCV inhibitors [abstract]. Hepatology 2006;44(Suppl 1):533A.
18. Nelson D, Pockros P, Godofsky E, et al. 84% end-of-treatment response (EOTR, week 48) achieved with R1626, peginterferon alfa 2a (40KD) and ribavirin for 4 weeks followed by the standard of care: Results of a phase 2a study in treatment-naïve HCV genotype 1 patients [abstract]. J Hepatol 2008;48(Suppl 2):S371.
19. Pockros P, Nelson D, Godofsky E, et al. High relapse rate seen at week 72 for patients treated with R1626 combination therapy. Hepatology 2008;48:1349–50.
20. Reddy R, Rodriguez-Torres M, Gane E, et al. Antiviral activity, pharmacokinetics, safety and tolerability of R7128, a novel nucleoside HCV RNA polymerase inhibitor, following multiple, ascending, oral doses in patients with HCV genotype 1 infection who have failed prior interferon therapy [abstract]. Hepatology 2007; 46(Suppl 1):862A.
21. Rodriguez-Torres M, Lalezari J, Gane E, et al. Potent antiviral response to the HCV nucleoside polymerase inhibitor R7128 for 28 days with Peg-IFN and ribavirin: subanalysis by race/ethnicity, eight and HCV genotype [abstract]. Hepatology 2008;48(Suppl):1160A.
22. Gane E, Rodriguez-Torres M, Nelson D, et al. Antiviral activity of the HCV nucleoside polymerase inhibitor R7128 in HCV genotype 2 and 3 prior non-responders; results of R7128 1500 mg BID with PEG-IFN and ribavirin for 28 days [abstract]. Hepatology 2008;48(Suppl 1):1024A.

23. Pharmasset and Roche obtain FDA consent to start a phase 2b study with R7128 in treatment naive HCV patients [press release]. Princeton (NJ): Pharmasset Inc.; 2009.
24. Cretton-Scott E, Perigaud C, Peyrottes S, et al. In vitro antiviral activity and pharmacology of IDX184, a novel and potent inhibitor of HCV replication [abstract]. J Hepatol 2008;48(Suppl 2):S220.
25. Accessed from Idenix website, Available at: www.indenix.com. Accessed February 14, 2009.
26. Carrol SS, Ludmerer S, Handt L, et al. Robust antiviral efficacy upon administration of a nucleoside analog to hepatitis C virus-infected chimpanzees. Antimicrob Agents Chemother 2009;53:926–34.
27. Kneteman NM, How AYM, Goa T, et al. HCV796: a selective nonstructural protein 5B polymerase inhibitor with potent anti-hepatitis C virus activity in vitro, in mice with chimeric human livers, and in humans infected with hepatitis C. Hepatology 2009;49:745–52.
28. Chandra P, Moyer L, Harper D, et al. Safety and pharmacokinetics of the non-nucleoside polymerase inhibitor, HCV-796: results of a randomized, double-blind, placebo-controlled, ascending single-dose study in healthy subjects. J Hepatol 2006;44(Suppl 2):S208–9.
29. Villano SA, Raible D, Harper D, et al. Antiviral activity of the non-nucleoside polymerase inhibitor, HCV-796, in combination with pegylated interferon alfa-2b in treatment-naïve patients with chronic HCV [abstract]. J Hepatol 2007;46:S24.
30. Villano S, Howe A, Raible D, et al. Analysis of HCV NS5B genetic variants following monotherapy with HCV-796, a non-nucleoside polymerase inhibitor in treatment naïve HCV-infected patients [abstract]. Hepatology 2006;44(Suppl 1):607A.
31. Press release. ViroPharma announces discontinuation of HCV-796 development. Exton (PA): ViroPharma; 2008.
32. Pockros PJ, Rodriguez-Torres M, Villano S, et al. A phase 2, randomized study of HCV-796 in combination with PEG-Intron plus Rebetol (RBV) versus PEG-Intron plus RBV in hepatitis C virus genotype 1 infection. European Association for the Study of Liver Disease Annual Meeting. Copenhagen, Denmark. April 22–29, 2009.
33. Erhardt A, Wedemeyer H, Benhamou Y, et al. Safety, pharmacokinetics and antiviral effects of BILB 1941, a novel HCV RNA polymerase, after 5 days oral treatment in patients with chronic hepatitis C [abstract]. J Hepatol 2007; 44(Suppl):S222.
34. Hammond JL, Rosario MC, Wagner F, et al. Antiviral activity of the HCV polymerase inhibitor PF-00868554 administered as monotherapy in HCV genotype 1 infected subjects [abstract]. Hepatology 2008;48(Suppl 1):267A.
35. Vliegen I, Paeshuyse J, Marbery E, et al. GS-9190, a novel substituted imidazopyridine analogue, is a potent inhibitor of hepatitis C virus replication in vitro and remains active against known drug resistant mutants [abstract]. Hepatology 2007;46(Suppl 1):855A.
36. Bavisotto L, Wang CC, Jacobson IM, et al. Antiviral, pharmacokinetic and safety data for GS 9190, a non-nucleoside HCV NS5b polymerase inhibitor, in a phase-1 trial in HCV genotype 1 infected subjects [abstract]. Hepatology 2007;46(Suppl 1):255A.
37. Cooper C, Lawitz EJ, Ghali P, et al. Antiviral activity of the non-nucleoside polymerase inhibitor, VCH-759, in chronic hepatitis C patients: results from a randomized double blind placebo controlled ascending multiple dose study [abstract]. Hepatology 2007;46(Suppl 1):864A.

38. Proulx L, Bourgault B, Chauret N, et al. Results of safety, tolerability and pharmacokinetic phase I study of VCH-916, a novel polymerase inhibitor for HCV, following single ascending doses in healthy volunteers. J Hepatol 2008;48;(Suppl 2):S320–1.
39. ANA598 (Anadys Pharmaceuticals). Available at: www.anadyspharma.com. Accessed February 14, 2009.
40. Lalezari J, Gane E, Rodriguez-Torres M, et al. Potent antiviral activity of the HCV nucleoside polymerase inhibitor R7128 with PEG-IFN and ribavirin: interim results of R7128 500 mg BID for 28 days [abstract]. J Hepatol 2008;48(Suppl 2):S29.
41. Sulkowski MS. Specific targeted antiviral therapy for hepatitis C. Curr Gastroenterol Rep 2007;9:5–13.

Caspase Inhibitors for the Treatment of Hepatitis C

Howard C. Masuoka, MD, PhD, Maria Eugenia Guicciardi, PhD, Gregory J. Gores, MD*

KEYWORDS

- Caspase inhibitors • Hepatitis C • Hepatic fibrogenesis
- Death receptors • Nonalcoholic steatohepatitis

APOPTOSIS AND LIVER INJURY

Apoptosis, a highly regulated form of cell death, represents the physiologic counterpart to mitosis, and together they provide the necessary regulation of cell number to maintain homeostatic cell turnover in adult organisms. Virtually any alteration in this balance, either toward excessive proliferation or excessive cell death, leads to the development of a pathologic condition. Apoptosis is also the most effective process employed by the immune system to eliminate mutated or infected cells. The apoptotic machinery can be activated externally by engagement of a subset of cell surface receptors belonging to the tumor necrosis factor (TNF) receptor superfamily, called death receptors, or internally by activation and release of mitochondrial proteins (**Fig. 1**). The common end point of both these pathways is the activation of a cascade of intracellular proteolytic enzymes called caspases (cysteinyl aspartate-specific proteases).

Caspases are cysteine proteases, which play a critical role in initiating and executing the apoptotic program by degrading several cellular components, resulting in the apoptotic phenotype. Apoptotic cells are then fragmented into small apoptotic bodies and engulfed by phagocytes. Engulfment of apoptotic bodies by stellate cells results in their activation, transformation to myofibroblasts, and increases their expression of collagen I.[1] In an analogous manner, phagocytosis of apoptotic bodies by Kupffer cells, the resident macrophages in the liver, increases their expression of death ligands for the death receptors.[2] Kupffer cell expression of death ligands may in turn promote further apoptosis of death receptor–expressing hepatocytes resulting

This work was supported by NIH Grants DK41876 to GJG, T3207198 for HCM and the Mayo Foundation.
Division of Gastroenterology and Hepatology, Miles and Shirley Fiterman Center for Digestive Diseases, College of Medicine, Mayo Clinic, 200 First Street SW, Rochester, MN 55905, USA
* Corresponding author.
E-mail address: gores.gregory@mayo.edu (G.J. Gores).

Clin Liver Dis 13 (2009) 467–475
doi:10.1016/j.cld.2009.05.010
liver.theclinics.com
1089-3261/09/$ – see front matter

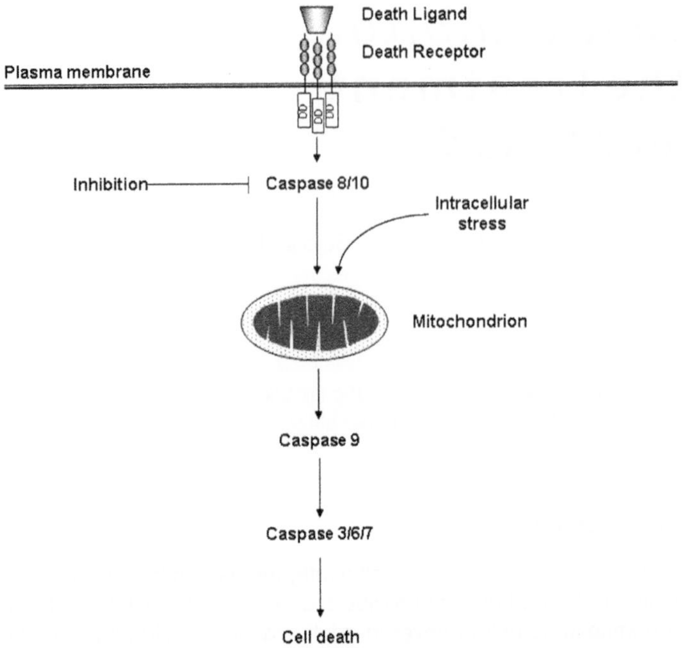

Fig. 1. The extrinsic pathway is initiated by the engagement of a death receptor by its cognate ligand, which results in initiator caspases 8 and 10. Activated initiator caspases cleave the BH3-only member of the Bcl-2 family Bid, which, in turn, causes mitochondrial dysfunction. The intrinsic pathway can be triggered by different intracellular stresses converging on the mitochondria. Both pathways lead to mitochondrial permeabilization with release of pro-apoptotic mitochondrial proteins, resulting in caspase 9 activation, and, subsequently, through a proteolytic cascade, activation of the effector caspases 3, 6 and 7, responsible for the degradation of numerous cellular components. Inhibition of caspases is an effective tool to block the extrinsic or death receptor pathway of cell death. Blocking caspase 9/3/6/7 will not prevent cell death as mitochondrial dysfunction, a lethal event, has already occurred.

in a feedforward mechanism whereby apoptosis begets more apoptosis. Thus, apoptosis promotes liver damage and fibrogenesis.[3] Inhibition of caspases often abrogates apoptosis. Caspases are synthesized as proenzymes and subsequently activated either by autocatalytic processing or by proteolytic cleavage by other caspases at an aspartate in the p1 position of the substrate. Several caspases have been identified, and, among them, caspases 2, 3, 6, 7, 8, 9, 10 have been demonstrated to play a role in apoptosis.[4]

CASPASE INHIBITION WILL NOT PROMOTE HEPATOCARCINOGENESIS

Clinicians may be concerned that inhibition of apoptosis promotes cancer. Therefore, this issue needs to be discussed. As mentioned above, there are 2 canonical pathways of apoptosis, death receptor (the so-called extrinsic pathway) versus non–death receptor (termed intrinsic pathway). The death receptor pathway is dependent on caspase 8 (see **Fig. 1**).[5] In the liver, the genetic absence of caspase 8 attenuates hepatitis in experimental models mediated by Fas or TNF-α.[6] The intrinsic or non-death receptor–mediated apoptosis is regulated by the B cell lymphoma 2 (Bcl-2) family of proteins and induces mitochondrial dysfunction resulting in activation of caspase 9, which in turn activates the effector caspase 3, 6, and 7. However, inhibition of caspase activation down stream of mitochondria only delays and does not prevent cell death.[7,8] Thus, pan-caspase inhibitors will likely only prevent cell death by death receptors. Animals with genetic deletions of death receptors do not develop spontaneous cancers.[9–11] Moreover, by blocking apoptosis, caspase inhibitors may actually reduce carcinogenesis in the liver, which requires cell turnover. Inhibition of apoptosis reduces cell turnover and in fact may be an antiapoptotic strategy. For example, apoptosis inhibition actually reduces hepatocarcinogenesis in a transgenic murine model of hepatitis B virus (HBV).[12] Therefore, caspase inhibitors in humans should only block death receptor–mediated apoptosis and should not promote cancer development.

HEPATITIS C VIRUS AND APOPTOSIS

Increased apoptosis is a hallmark of active hepatitis C infection, and the level of hepatocyte apoptosis correlates with the histologic activity grade.[13] It has been suggested that hepatocytes apoptosis may be a mechanism for viral shedding and thus inhibition of apoptosis could ameliorate hepatitis C.[14] Hepatitis C virus (HCV) infection has been shown to influence the death receptor–mediated pathway and the mitochondrial apoptotic pathway.[15] Consistently, increased caspase-cleaved products of cytokeratin-18 (CK-18), the major intermediate filament in hepatocytes, are present in serum and liver biopsies of HCV-infected patients compared with healthy controls, demonstrating that caspases are activated during HCV infection.[16] Moreover, caspase activation correlates with the degree of inflammatory liver injury, that is, necroinflammatory activity, in chronic hepatitis C infection.[16,17] The mechanism through which this increase in apoptosis is mediated is still being defined, but several lines of evidence suggest that it is primarily immune-mediated. Although HCV itself has mild cytopathic effects on the infected host cells, the extensive tissue damage associated with viral hepatitis is generally the result of host immune response to the viral antigen. During viral hepatitis, specific classes of cytotoxic T lymphocytes (CTL) recognize and kill viral antigen-presenting, HCV-infected hepatocytes to clear the virus from the liver. This process causes the initial liver damage, which is exacerbated by the influx of antigen-nonspecific inflammatory cells. The antigen-primed CTL and CD8+ T lymphocytes directly kill HCV-infected hepatocytes by cell–cell contact, and release of cytotoxic or antiviral cytokines such as interferon-γ (IFN-γ) and TNF-α. The killing occurs by apoptosis, as demonstrated by the presence of apoptotic bodies, once referred to as Councilman bodies, in close proximity to infiltrating CD8+ T lymphocytes in the liver of patients with viral hepatitis.[13] Death receptor–mediated apoptosis, in particular, is critical in HCV associated liver injury. Immune effector cells express the death ligands, Fas ligand, and TNF-related apoptosis-inducing ligand (TRAIL), and secrete TNF-α. Consistently, upregulation of the main death receptors and their ligands has been described in HCV infection.[13,18]

If a death receptor is engaged by its cognate ligand (Fas ligand, TRAIL, or TNF-α), a series of conformational changes occurs that leads to the recruitment of intracellular cytoplasmic adaptor molecules, which provides a platform for recruitment and activation of the initiator caspases 8 or 10. The activated initiator caspases, in turn, start a proteolytic cascade resulting in activation of other caspases referred to as effector caspases (caspase 3, 6 and 7), either by direct cleavage of the effector caspase or indirectly by cleavage and activation of other substrates (ie, the Bcl-2 protein Bid), which promotes mitochondrial permeabilization and release of caspase-activating factors (ie, cytochrome *c*) (see **Fig. 1**). Among the death receptors, the Fas/FasL (CD95/CD95L) system plays the most important pathogenic role in this process.[19] Upregulation of Fas in hepatocytes and FasL induction in T lymphocytes have been observed in the liver of patients with chronic hepatitis C, and directly correlate with disease activity such as periportal and intralobular inflammation.[20–24] In addition to Fas, other death receptors have been implicated in the pathogenesis of HCV-mediated liver injury. TNF-α expression is increased in the liver of HCV-infected patients, and HCV-specific CTLs have been shown to secrete TNF-α in vitro.[25,26] Moreover, TNF-α and the soluble form of its receptor, TNF-receptor 1 (TNF-R1), are often elevated in the serum of patients with HCV infection, especially during fulminant hepatitis, suggesting this system may play a more important role in acute inflammation than in chronic hepatitic.[27,28] TRAIL is also increased in hepatocytes from patients with chronic hepatitis C,[29] and expression of TRAIL in CD8+ T cells and CD68+ macrophages has been reported to be increased in the immediate vicinity of apoptotic hepatocytes in HCV-infected liver.[30] TRAIL expression is increased in chronic hepatitis C independent of the extent of lymphocyte infiltration.[31,32] Unlike FasL, TRAIL induces apoptosis only in infected cells, demonstrating that other cytokines or perhaps the virus itself sensitizes hepatocytes to TRAIL-mediated apoptosis.[33] It is not clear whether Fas or TRAIL expression is mainly regulated by virus-specific proteins or by inflammatory cytokines, such as interleukin-1 (IL-1), generated after the first immune response. In general, the role of the individual HCV proteins in apoptosis remains controversial, as multiple proteins encoded by the HCV genome have been demonstrated to have pro- or antiapoptotic effects.[34] Because of the long-time unavailability of tissue culture systems or animal models suitable for HCV replication, most of these data have been generated in studies employing either in vitro overexpression systems or transgenic animal models, which do not adequately reproduce the clinical situation in HCV-infected patients; the viral proteins are usually present at low levels, and therefore the results must be interpreted cautiously. However, the recent establishment of an efficient cell culture system that hosts the complete viral life cycle in human hepatocyte-derived target cells has allowed the study of HCV-host interaction and apoptosis in a more appropriate model.[35,36] Using this model, recent studies have demonstrated that HCV infection renders hepatocytes sensitive to TRAIL-induced apoptosis, suggesting an essential contribution of the mitochondrial pathway of apoptosis in HCV-mediated sensitization to TRAIL.[18,30,37] Caspase-dependent apoptosis of HCV-specific CD8+ T cells has also been demonstrated in acute and chronic HCV infection and may play a role in preventing an effective T cell response and viral persistence.[38–40]

Chronic HCV infection is characterized by variable degrees of hepatic inflammation, damage and fibrosis with progressive risk of developing liver cirrhosis and hepatocellular carcinoma. Hepatocytes apoptosis during HCV infection might directly promote liver fibrosis by activation of stellate cells and Kupffer cells.[3] Engulfment of apoptotic bodies by stellate cells in vitro increases expression of collagen and transforming growth factor β (TGF-β) in a cell culture model.[1] Similarly, Kupffer cell engulfment of apoptotic bodies promotes inflammation and fibrogenesis.[2] Therefore, inhibition of caspase activation and apoptosis during HCV may be beneficial not only to reduce liver damage but also to prevent the onset of liver fibrosis.

CASPASE INHIBITORS IN PRECLINICAL STUDIES OF LIVER DISEASE

Treatment with the pan-caspase inhibitor ZVAD-fmk resulted in decreased mortality in the rat massive hepatectomy model of acute liver failure.[41] Infusion of the pan-caspase inhibitor IDN-6556 ((3-{2-[(2-tert-butyl-phenylaminooxalyl)-amino]-propionylamino}-4-oxo-5-(2,3,5,6-tetrafluoro-phenoxy)-pentanoic acid)) has also been shown to reduce ischemia-reperfusion injury in rodent models.[42–44] IDN-6556 has been shown to be effective in reducing transaminase elevation and apoptosis in rodent models of acute liver injury.[45] More importantly, a caspase inhibitor also reduced hepatic fibrosis in the bile duct ligated mouse.[46] This latter study provided solid preclinical data indicating that caspase inhibitors can mitigate hepatic fibrogenesis in addition to simply reducing the magnitude of apoptosis. Deletion of the death receptor Fas or the death ligand TRAIL also attenuate hepatic fibrogenesis in the bile duct ligated animal. Thus, the data to date indicate that inhibition of death receptor–mediated apoptosis attenuates liver injury in preclinical models.

CASPASE INHIBITORS IN HUMAN LIVER INJURY

Data employing caspase inhibitors in humans are scant. Caspase inhibitors for human use were developed by IDUN Pharmaceuticals, Gilead Sciences, Inc, and Vertex Pharmaceuticals. However, only 1 proof of concept trial has been performed in patients with HCV.[47] This study employed IDN-6556, which was developed by IDUN Pharmaceuticals, later purchased by Pfizer. IDN-6556 is an irreversible pan-caspase inhibitor. IDN-6556 also inhibits caspase 1, which has been implicated in inflammation; thus, the drug may also inhibit inflammation in addition to blocking apoptosis. The study design was a multicenter, double-blind, placebo-controlled, dose-ranging study with only a 14-day dosing period. At the time of the study design and implementation, long-term animal toxicity data were not available, so the FDA appropriately limited the duration of the study. A total of 105 patients were enrolled in the study; 79 received active drug, 80 patients had chronic hepatitis C, and 25 had other liver diseases including nonalcoholic steatohepatitis (NASH), hepatitis B, primary biliary cirrhosis (PBC), and primary sclerosing cholangitis (PSC). The does of IDN-6556 in the study ranged from 5 to 400 mg orally on a daily basis. In the HCV patient population, all doses of IDN-6556 significantly lowered alanine aminotransferase (ALT) and aspartate aminotransferase (AST) (**Fig. 2**). Declines in aminotransferase activity were also observed in 4 patients with NASH (**Fig. 3**). No adverse reactions to the drug were noted in this 2-week study. Mean HCV RNA levels were not altered by drug administration compared with baseline values. Thus, oral IDN-6556 does lower serum aminotransferase activity in HCV patients. Longer-term studies will be required to assess the potential effects of IDN-6556 on liver inflammation and fibrosis.

A human trial with IDN-6556 was also conducted in organ preservation injury.[48] What was reported from the study was a post hoc analysis of a Phase II, multicenter, randomized, placebo-controlled, double-blinded, parallel group study. Subjects were assigned to 4 treatment groups: Group 1 (organ storage/flush, placebo-recipient, placebo); Group 2 (organ storage/flush, 15 μg/mL-recipient, placebo); Group 3 (organ storage/flush, 5 μg/mL-recipient, 0.5 mg/kg); and Group 4 (organ storage/flush, 15 μg/mL-recipient, 0.5 mg/kg). Terminal deoxynucleotide transferase-mediated dUTP nick-end labeling (TUNEL) assay and caspase 3/7 immunohistochemistry were performed to measure liver apoptosis. Liver injury was assessed by serum AST/ALT determinations. Serum markers of the CK18Asp396 (M30) neo-epitope (a cleavage product of caspase 3 and therefore a biomarker for hepatocyte apoptosis) were reduced in all groups receiving drug compared with placebo. However, serum AST/ALT levels were only consistently reduced in Group 2 (drug exposed to organ only). As to why the caspase inhibitor was not additive when also given to the recipient, is likely to be explained by the increase in neutrophils accumulating in the liver of those

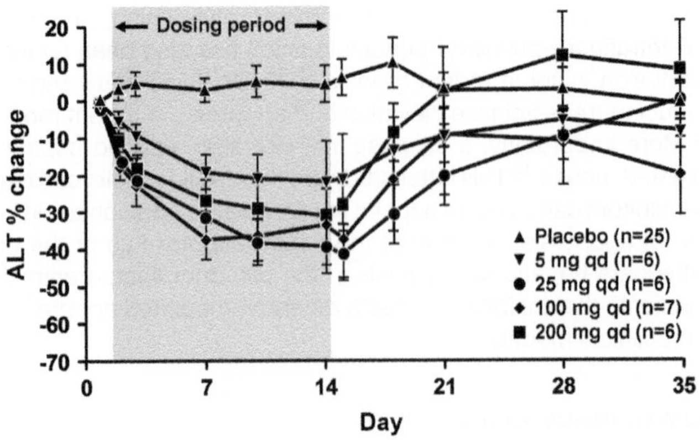

Fig. 2. Patients received IDN-6556 orally once a day at the dose indicated. Changes in serum ALT values are expressed as percent change from baseline. QD dosing indicates once a day drug administration. Data are expressed as the means ± standard error of the mean (SEM). (*Reprinted from* Pockros PJ, Schiff ER, Shiffman ML, et al. Oral IDN-6556, an antiapoptotic caspase inhibitor, may lower aminotransferase activity in patients with chronic hepatitis C. Hepatology 2007;46(2):326; with permission.)

recipients receiving active drug. Perhaps inhibition of neutrophil apoptosis permitted their accumulation in the liver following ischemia/reperfusion injury. The neutrophils would then further injure the liver. These observations illustrate the complexity of inhibiting apoptosis in multiple cell types in this form of liver damage. Nonetheless, IDN-6556, when administered in cold storage and flush solutions during liver transplantation, seems to offer local therapeutic protection against cold ischemia/warm reperfusion liver injury.

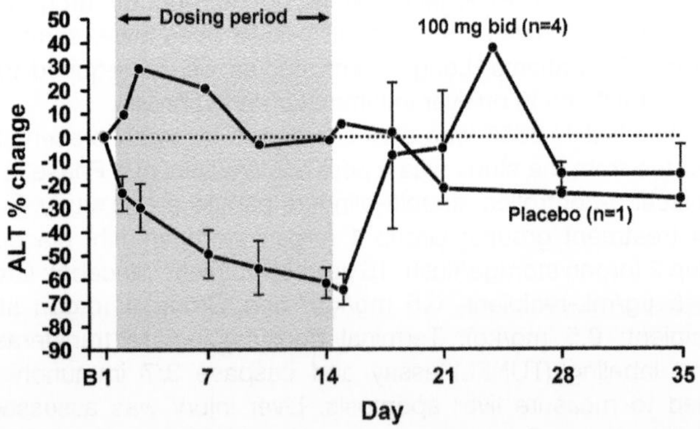

Fig. 3. Four patients with NASH were treated with IDN-6556 at a dose of 100 mg orally twice a day. Changes in the serum ALT values are expressed as a percent change from baseline. Results are the mean ± SEM in 4 patients. (*Reprinted from* Pockros PJ, Schiff ER, Shiffman ML, et al. Oral IDN-6556, an antiapoptotic caspase inhibitor, may lower aminotransferase activity in patients with chronic hepatitis C. Hepatology 2007;46(2):327; with permission.)

SUMMARY

Several preclinical and early clinical studies suggest a potential benefit for caspase inhibitors in liver injury. However, significant methodologic issues including small sample size, short follow-up, and use of surrogate markers, is present in all the current studies. In particular, none of these agents has been shown to consistently decrease the critical outcomes of mortality or time to transplant. Although the results are intriguing, additional carefully designed studies with adequate methodology, patient sample size, and follow-up need to be performed before any of these medications may be recommended for the treatment of hepatitis C. Nonetheless, caspase inhibitors are extremely promising hepatoprotective agents and their further study is strongly encouraged.

REFERENCES

1. Canbay A, Taimr P, Torok N, et al. Apoptotic body engulfment by a human stellate cell line is profibrogenic. Lab Invest 2003;83(5):655–63.
2. Canbay A, Feldstein AE, Higuchi H, et al. Kupffer cell engulfment of apoptotic bodies stimulates death ligand and cytokine expression. Hepatology 2003; 38(5):1188–98.
3. Canbay A, Friedman S, Gores GJ. Apoptosis: the nexus of liver injury and fibrosis. Hepatology 2004;39(2):273–8.
4. Thornberry NA, Lazebnik Y. Caspases: enemies within. Science 1998;281(5381): 1312–6.
5. Zender L, Hutker S, Liedtke C, et al. Caspase 8 small interfering RNA prevents acute liver failure in mice. Proc Natl Acad Sci U S A 2003;100(13):7797–802.
6. Kaufmann T, Jost PJ, Pellegrini M, et al. Fatal hepatitis mediated by tumor necrosis factor TNFalpha requires caspase-8 and involves the BH3-only proteins Bid and Bim. Immunity 2009;30(1):56–66.
7. Chen J, Nagayama T, Jin K, et al. Induction of caspase-3-like protease may mediate delayed neuronal death in the hippocampus after transient cerebral ischemia. J Neurosci 1998;18(13):4914–28.
8. Strobel T, Swanson L, Korsmeyer S, et al. BAX enhances paclitaxel-induced apoptosis through a p53-independent pathway. Proc Natl Acad Sci U S A 1996;93(24):14094–9.
9. Adachi M, Suematsu S, Kondo T, et al. Targeted mutation in the Fas gene causes hyperplasia in peripheral lymphoid organs and liver. Nat Genet 1995;11(3): 294–300.
10. Pfeffer K, Matsuyama T, Kundig TM, et al. Mice deficient for the 55 kd tumor necrosis factor receptor are resistant to endotoxic shock, yet succumb to *L. monocytogenes* infection. Cell 1993;73(3):457–67.
11. Yue HH, Diehl GE, Winoto A. Loss of TRAIL-R does not affect thymic or intestinal tumor development in p53 and adenomatous polyposis coli mutant mice. Cell Death Differ 2005;12(1):94–7.
12. Nakamoto Y, Kaneko S, Fan H, et al. Prevention of hepatocellular carcinoma development associated with chronic hepatitis by anti-fas ligand antibody therapy. J Exp Med 2002;196(8):1105–11.
13. Calabrese F, Pontisso P, Pettenazzo E, et al. Liver cell apoptosis in chronic hepatitis C correlates with histological but not biochemical activity or serum HCV-RNA levels. Hepatology 2000;31(5):1153–9.
14. Kountouras J, Zavos C, Chatzopoulos D. Apoptosis in hepatitis C. J Viral Hepat 2003;10(5):335–42.

15. Mengshol JA, Golden-Mason L, Rosen HR. Mechanisms of disease: HCV-induced liver injury. Nat Clin Pract Gastroenterol Hepatol 2007;4(11):622–34.
16. Bantel H, Lugering A, Heidemann J, et al. Detection of apoptotic caspase activation in sera from patients with chronic HCV infection is associated with fibrotic liver injury. Hepatology 2004;40(5):1078–87.
17. Bantel H, Lugering A, Poremba C, et al. Caspase activation correlates with the degree of inflammatory liver injury in chronic hepatitis C virus infection. Hepatology 2001;34(4 Pt 1):758–67.
18. Volkmann X, Fischer U, Bahr MJ, et al. Increased hepatotoxicity of tumor necrosis factor-related apoptosis-inducing ligand in diseased human liver. Hepatology 2007;46(5):1498–508.
19. Hayashi N, Mita E. Involvement of Fas system-mediated apoptosis in pathogenesis of viral hepatitis. J Viral Hepat 1999;6(5):357–65.
20. Mochizuki K, Hayashi N, Hiramatsu N, et al. Fas antigen expression in liver tissues of patients with chronic hepatitis B. J Hepatol 1996;24(1):1–7.
21. Luo KX, Zhu YF, Zhang LX, et al. In situ investigation of Fas/FasL expression in chronic hepatitis B infection and related liver diseases. J Viral Hepat 1997;4(5):303–7.
22. Galle PR, Hofmann WJ, Walczak H, et al. Involvement of the CD95 (APO-1/Fas) receptor and ligand in liver damage. J Exp Med 1995;182(5):1223–30.
23. Hiramatsu N, Hayashi N, Katayama K, et al. Immunohistochemical detection of Fas antigen in liver tissue of patients with chronic hepatitis C. Hepatology 1994;19(6):1354–9.
24. Yoneyama K, Goto T, Miura K, et al. The expression of Fas and Fas ligand, and the effects of interferon in chronic liver diseases with hepatitis C virus. Hepatol Res 2002;24(4):327–37.
25. Ando K, Hiroishi K, Kaneko T, et al. Perforin, Fas/Fas ligand, and TNF-alpha pathways as specific and bystander killing mechanisms of hepatitis C virus-specific human CTL. J Immunol 1997;158(11):5283–91.
26. Gonzalez-Amaro R, Garcia-Monzon C, Garcia-Buey L, et al. Induction of tumor necrosis factor alpha production by human hepatocytes in chronic viral hepatitis. J Exp Med 1994;179(3):841–8.
27. Bantel H, Schulze-Osthoff K. Apoptosis in hepatitis C virus infection. Cell Death Differ 2003;10(Suppl 1):S48–58.
28. Tokushige K, Yamaguchi N, Ikeda I, et al. Significance of soluble TNF receptor-I in acute-type fulminant hepatitis. Am J Gastroenterol 2000;95(8):2040–6.
29. Mundt B, Kuhnel F, Zender L, et al. Involvement of TRAIL and its receptors in viral hepatitis. FASEB J 2003;17(1):94–6.
30. Lan L, Gorke S, Rau SJ, et al. Hepatitis C virus infection sensitizes human hepatocytes to TRAIL-induced apoptosis in a caspase 9-dependent manner. J Immunol 2008;181(7):4926–35.
31. Zheng SJ, Wang P, Tsabary G, et al. Critical roles of TRAIL in hepatic cell death and hepatic inflammation. J Clin Invest 2004;113(1):58–64.
32. Piekarska A, Kubiak R, Omulecka A, et al. Expression of tumour necrosis factor-related apoptosis-inducing ligand and caspase-3 in relation to grade of inflammation and stage of fibrosis in chronic hepatitis C. Histopathology 2007;51(5):597–604.
33. Mundt B, Wirth T, Zender L, et al. Tumour necrosis factor related apoptosis inducing ligand (TRAIL) induces hepatic steatosis in viral hepatitis and after alcohol intake. Gut 2005;54(11):1590–6.
34. Fischer R, Baumert T, Blum HE. Hepatitis C virus infection and apoptosis. World J Gastroenterol 2007;13(36):4865–72.

35. Lindenbach BD, Evans MJ, Syder AJ, et al. Complete replication of hepatitis C virus in cell culture. Science 2005;309(5734):623–6.
36. Wakita T, Pietschmann T, Kato T, et al. Production of infectious hepatitis C virus in tissue culture from a cloned viral genome. Nat Med 2005;11(7):791–6.
37. Chou AH, Tsai HF, Wu YY, et al. Hepatitis C virus core protein modulates TRAIL-mediated apoptosis by enhancing Bid cleavage and activation of mitochondria apoptosis signaling pathway. J Immunol 2005;174(4):2160–6.
38. Radziewicz H, Ibegbu CC, Hon H, et al. Impaired hepatitis C virus (HCV)-specific effector CD8+ T cells undergo massive apoptosis in the peripheral blood during acute HCV infection and in the liver during the chronic phase of infection. J Virol 2008;82(20):9808–22.
39. Radziewicz H, Ibegbu CC, Fernandez ML, et al. Liver-infiltrating lymphocytes in chronic human hepatitis C virus infection display an exhausted phenotype with high levels of PD-1 and low levels of CD127 expression. J Virol 2007;81(6): 2545–53.
40. Toubi E, Kessel A, Goldstein L, et al. Enhanced peripheral T-cell apoptosis in chronic hepatitis C virus infection: association with liver disease severity. J Hepatol 2001;35(6):774–80.
41. Yoshida N, Iwata H, Yamada T, et al. Improvement of the survival rate after rat massive hepatectomy due to the reduction of apoptosis by caspase inhibitor. J Gastroenterol Hepatol 2007;22(11):2015–21.
42. Natori S, Selzner M, Valentino KL, et al. Apoptosis of sinusoidal endothelial cells occurs during liver preservation injury by a caspase-dependent mechanism. Transplantation 1999;68(1):89–96.
43. Natori S, Higuchi H, Contreras P, et al. The caspase inhibitor IDN-6556 prevents caspase activation and apoptosis in sinusoidal endothelial cells during liver preservation injury. Liver Transpl 2003;9(3):278–84.
44. Hoglen NC, Anselmo DM, Katori M, et al. A caspase inhibitor IDN-6556, ameliorates early hepatic injury in an ex vivo rat model of warm and cold ischemia. Liver Transpl 2007;13(3):361–6.
45. Hoglen NC, Chen LS, Fisher CD, et al. Characterization of IDN-6556 (3-[2-(2-tert-butyl-phenylaminooxalyl)-amino]-propionylamino]-4-oxo-5-(2,3,5,6-tetrafluoro-phenoxy)-pentanoic acid): a liver-targeted caspase inhibitor. J Pharmacol Exp Ther 2004;309(2):634–40.
46. Canbay A, Feldstein A, Baskin-Bey E, et al. The caspase inhibitor IDN-6556 attenuates hepatic injury and fibrosis in the bile duct ligated mouse. J Pharmacol Exp Ther 2004;308(3):1191–6.
47. Pockros PJ, Schiff ER, Shiffman ML, et al. Oral IDN-6556, an antiapoptotic caspase inhibitor, may lower aminotransferase activity in patients with chronic hepatitis C. Hepatology 2007;46(2):324–9.
48. Baskin-Bey ES, Washburn K, Feng S, et al. Clinical trial of the pan-caspase inhibitor, IDN-6556, in human liver preservation injury. Am J Transplant 2007;7(1): 218–25.

Monoclonal and Polyclonal Antibodies Against the HCV Envelope Proteins

Heshaam M. Mir, MD[a,b], Aybike Birerdinc, PhD[b],
Zobair M. Younossi, MD, MPH[a,b,*]

KEYWORDS

- Monoclonal • Polyclonal • Antibodies
- Hepatitis C • Treatment

Hepatitis C Virus (HCV) causes significant health problems worldwide. Development of an effective drug for the prevention and management of HCV has been hindered by the ability of this virus to remain latent and its ability to mutate, which gives rise to numerous genetically distinct strains.[1,2] In fact, the United States Centers for Disease Control and Prevention (CDC) rates HCV as the most common chronic blood-borne infection.[3] Furthermore, 75% to 85% of individuals initially infected with the HCV become chronically infected, with 20% progressing to advanced liver disease. Because of the tremendous disease burden of HCV, it is the most common indication for liver transplantation. Although liver transplant can address cirrhosis and its complications, post-transplant reoccurrence is universal and is even more difficult to prevent or treat successfully than patients treated in the pretransplant setting.[4,5]

The ability of HCV to constantly mutate is partly responsible for the high rates of HCV-related chronicity and has resulted in several different genotypes, subtypes, and quasispecies with slightly different genomic sequences.[5] This genetic diversity has thwarted efforts to produce vaccines, neutralizing antibodies and is, at least partly, responsible for the difficulty in finding a universal cure for the HCV virus.[5]

The current standard treatment of HCV is associated with a sustained virologic response of 50% to 55%. However, this drug combination (pegylated interferon-a and ribavirin) is fraught with numerous side effects and adherence issues.[2,5] Furthermore, the efficacy of this combination for the most common HCV genotype

[a] Center for Liver Diseases, Inova Fairfax Hospital, 3300 Gallows Road, Falls Church, VA 22042, USA
[b] Betty and Guy Beatty Center for Integrated Research, Inova Health System, Falls Church, VA 22042, USA
* Corresponding author. Betty and Guy Beatty Center for Integrated Research, Inova Health System, 3300 Gallows Road, Claude Moore Building, 3rd Floor, Falls Church, Virginia 22042.
E-mail address: zobair.younossi@inova.org (Z.M. Younossi).

Clin Liver Dis 13 (2009) 477–486
doi:10.1016/j.cld.2009.05.011

(genotypes 1) is lower.[5] In addition, this combination has a poor response rate in individuals who have already failed a course of treatment.[5]

An important step forward in HCV treatment is the availability of a new culture system, which is providing insights into the biology of HCV and opportunities for identifying and pursuing methods that could lead to the discovery of novel antiviral therapies for HCV.[2] The novel therapeutics in the pipeline include the development of monoclonal and polyclonal antibodies. Other very promising novel agents include specifically targeted antiviral therapy for hepatitis C (STAT-C) and other treatment strategies, summarized in this issue of *Clinics in Liver Disease*. In theory, these therapeutic options have the potential to be much more effective and are associated with fewer and less serious side effects than the current treatment combination.

Immunoglobulin G (IgG) collected from HCV-positive patients has been tested against HCV and shown to have transient protective activity against the virus in chimpanzees.[6] Two other monoclonal antibodies exhibit preventive activity against a wide range of HCV strains in animals or humans.[7–9] These and several other breakthrough drugs still in the preclinical stages of development show great potential in the drive for effective drugs and vaccines against HCV infection.[7,10,11]

VIROLOGY

Life Cycle

The HCV viral polyprotein is processed by a combination of virally encoded and cellular proteases. This process produces 10 structural and nonstructural proteins. The structural proteins, which are mostly enveloped glycoproteins, constitute the bulk of the viral structure, whereas the nonstructural proteins perform catalytic functions. E1 and E2 are believed to be the most important structural proteins.[12] To a large extent, they constitute the virion structure and are believed to facilitate viral entry and the subsequent fusion with the host cell membrane. Once inside the host cell, the HCV releases its nucleocapsid into the host cell's cytoplasm, thus initiating viral polyprotein translation within the replication complex.[12] The RNA-dependent RNA polymerase (RdRp), encoded by nonstructural protein 5 (NS5) and the NS3, initiates viral RNA maturation and encapsulation occurs within the endoplasmic reticulum. The viral nucleocapsids are then enveloped and maturate inside the Golgi apparatus before finally being released into the pericellular space through exocytosis (**Fig. 1**).[12]

Mechanism of Cell Entry and Fusion

The early process of attachment and entry of HCV into the host cell involves 2 groups of proteins, the HCV structural proteins and receptor molecules at the surface of the target cells, whereas fusion is mediated by RNA-dependent RNA polymerase (RdRp) and NS3 of the virus. The structure of the E1 and E2 enveloped glycoproteins of HCV may facilitate attachment and entry into target cells. In fact, these glycoproteins have a molecular weight of 33 to 35 and 70 to 72 kilodaltons, respectively, and assemble noncovalent heterodimers. They are also believed to be highly glycosylated, containing up to 5 and 11 glycosylation sites each and with several hypervariable regions, especially in E2.[13]

The first step toward cellular attachment is believed to be initiated by E2 through its interaction with one or more components of the receptor complex. Some of the receptors on the cellular surface that are believed to constitute this "receptor complex" include glycosaminoglycans, CD81, Claudin-1, and scavenger receptor B type I (SR-BI). E2 is believed to participate in cellular attachment by the interaction between hypervariable 1 (HPVR1), a region of E2 that has positively charged residues at specific

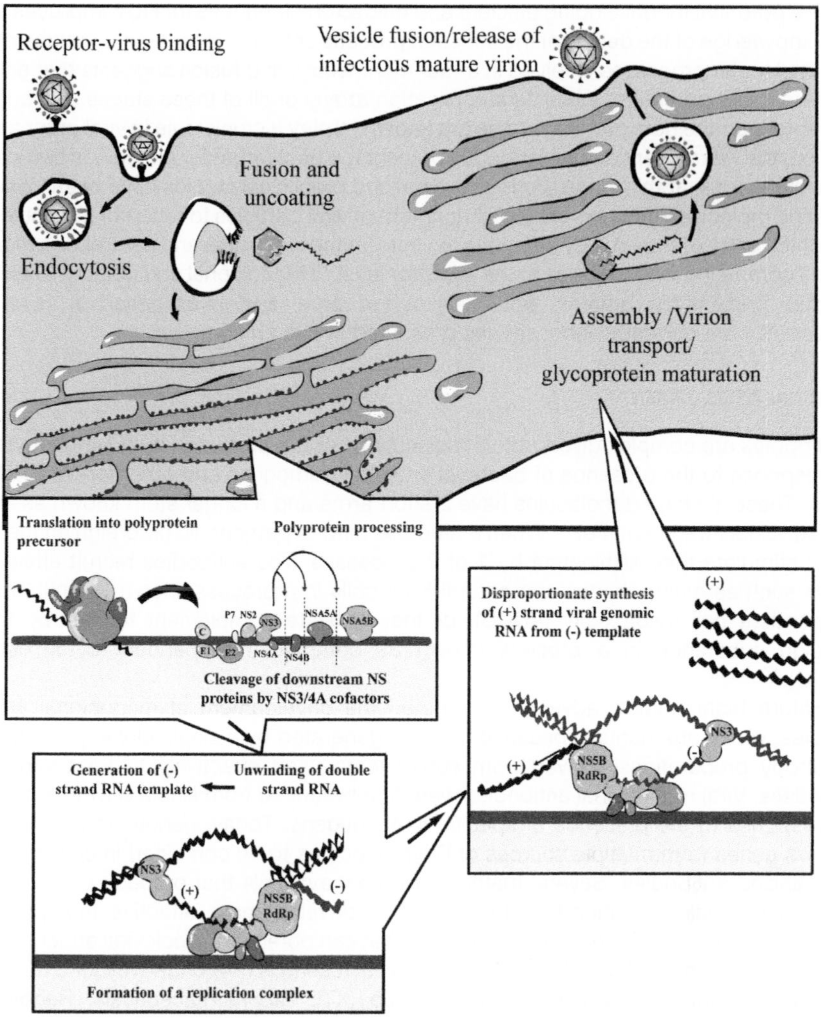

Fig. 1. The life cycle of hepatitis C virus. (*Data from* Pawlotsky J, Chaveliez S, McHutchison JG. The hepatitis C virus life cycle as a target for new antiviral therapies. Gastroenterology 2007;132:1979–98.)

sequence positions, and the negatively charged molecules on the surface of target cells. Human serum seems to facilitate the infection of liver cells, probably through the interaction between high-density lipoproteins (HDL), HVR1, and the SR-BI.[13–15]

After attachment, viral entry is believed to be pH-dependent and mediated by clathrin-dependent endocytosis, and the entry is followed by fusion within an acidic endosomal compartment.[15] Although the actual process and peptides that mediate the fusion process are still unclear, sequence analysis suggests the presence of fusion peptide in the ectodomain of E1, and the transmembrane domains of E1 and E2 have been shown to play crucial roles in fusion. Once fusion is achieved, the viral nucleocapsid is released into the cytoplasm of the affected cell and the process of replication and maturation continues.[12]

The potential for developing efficient and efficacious therapies for HCV improves as our knowledge of the details of the infection process unfolds. For example, insight into the molecular processes involved in attachment, entry, and fusion suggests that antibodies could potentially inhibit viral replication at any or all of these stages. Because receptors on the host cell membrane are known to play a crucial role in viral entry and fusion, the attachment and entry stages present the best target for antibodies that can attack the virus at this stage. Various clinical and preclinical studies have been investigating molecules that prevent the attachment of viral particles to receptor molecules, or inhibit entry of the virus by attaching to viral surface structures and neutralizing them or by competing with the virus at the receptor level.[16] Monoclonal and polyclonal antibodies present the greatest potentials in this area, and investigation of several antibodies are currently underway, as presented in this article.

CLINICAL DEVELOPMENT

Antibodies are complex glycoprotein molecules that are produced by B lymphocytes in response to the presence of bacterial and viral pathogens and other foreign particles. These Y-shaped molecules have 2 short arms and a longer stem known as the crystallizable fragment (Fc).[17] When antibodies bind to pathogenic or foreign antigens they stimulate their elimination by 1 of 2 processes. The antibodies recruit effector cells such as macrophages and natural killer cells in a process known as antibody-dependent cell cytotoxicity (ADCC), or they activate complement to destroy the foreign substance in a process known as complement-dependent cytotoxicity (CDC).[17]

Before technological advances promoted the development of monoclonal antibodies, which are identical because they are generated by a single clone, polyclonal antibody preparations derived from serum were used effectively to treat various diseases. Viral monoclonal antibodies were first produced from single B lymphocytes in response to the presence of specific viral antigens. Today, genetic manipulation allows genes from multiple sources of B lymphocytes to be combined in chimeric or humanized antibodies. Several methods are now available that produce completely human monoclonal antibodies. In the bid to develop more effective therapy for HCV, polyclonal and monoclonal antibodies that can potentially block viral attachment or entry are being tested.[17] Phase I and II clinical testing is now underway for 3 monoclonal antibodies: HCV AB68, HCV AB6865 (XTL Biopharmaceuticals, Rehovot, Israel), Bavituximab (Peregrine Pharmaceuticals, Tustin, CA); and a polyclonal antibody, Civacir (NABI Biopharmaceuticals, Boca Raton, FL).[8,10,18,19] Some of the results from these studies are summarized later.

HCV AB68 and HCV AB6865

AB68 is a human monoclonal antibody that has high binding affinity for the E2 envelope protein of HCV. The antibody was generated by immortalizing peripheral blood mononuclear cells obtained from the blood of donor patients who tested positive to HCV. AB68 belongs to the immunoglobulin subtype 1 (IgG1). Its binding power with E2 is indicated by the presence of 4 amino acids at the C-terminal of HVR 1 and an unclear number of E2 amino acids, which specify the epitope recognized by AB68. The antibody immunoprecipitates HCV RNA in the blood serum of infected patients with HCV genotypes 1a/1b, 2a/2c, and 3a. Immunohistochemistry shows that the antibody specifically labels the cytoplasm of liver cells from HCV-infected liver fragments. These studies confirm that AB68 recognizes the HCV virus in infected cells. Preclinical testing shows that AB68 inhibits HCV infection in the HCV-Trimera mouse model, as it reduced the percentage of infected animals and reduced the viral load in animals treated with the antibody after HCV infection.

The tolerability and efficacy of this antibody has since been tested in a randomized, double-blind, placebo-controlled, dose-escalation clinical study.[18] This study was performed in different centers and divided into parts I and II. Subjects were eligible for the study if they were 18 to 65 years of age, undergoing liver transplant due to HCV infection, and were HCV-positive as measured by HCV RNA level above the local limit for at least a year. The subjects in part I of the study (n = 12) received 1 of 3 doses (20, 40, or 80 mg), whereas those in part II received 1 of 3 higher doses (120, 240, or 480 mg). For each dose, subjects were randomized to treatment with AB68 or placebo in a 3:1 ratio. Subjects in part I received the study drug intravenously once during the anhepatic phase, once postoperatively, once after admission into the intensive care unit, and once daily for another 6 days. After the sixth day, the subjects in part I received the study drug once weekly for the next 3 weeks and then every 4 weeks for the next 8 weeks. Subjects in part II received the higher doses of the study drug or placebo in 4 installments. The first installment occurred 2 hours after the anhepatic phase began, and the second, third, and fourth installments were administered over approximately 8 hours per dose beginning with the time of liver reperfusion. Subjects in this group then received the study drug or placebo daily for the next 6 days, weekly for 3 weeks, and at 2-week intervals for 8 weeks.

The investigators report a difference of almost 1 log HCV RNA units post liver transplantation, especially in the 120- to 240-mg dose group. The serum levels in subjects receiving this dose were 50 to 200 μg/ml higher than that of subjects receiving placebo. Also, the median serum level of HCV RNA dropped from baseline with all dosages immediately after liver transplantation. The serum levels of HCV RNA were initially reduced by 1.8 to 2.4 log in the 120- to 240-mg dose group, but this difference was lost after 7 days when the dosing frequency was reduced. The drug was well tolerated, with no reports of fatal or severe adverse effect in any dosage groups. In fact, the investigators report that the occurrence of nonfatal serious adverse effects was higher in the placebo group (60%) compared with an average (42%) for all the treatment groups.[18]

The investigators suggest that the observed coincident increase in anti-E2 antibodies in the sera of subjects receiving the study drug and the decrease in HCV RNA levels implies that the dose-related changes in HCV RNA concentration were induced by the administered AB68. They conclude that AB68 is effective against HCV infection with few adverse effects. However, the investigators point out the necessity for studies evaluating the effect of more frequent daily dosing on sustaining the reduced viral load observed in this study.

Another phase 1b clinical study was performed in 2007 to evaluate the efficacy of AB68 in patients with chronic hepatitis C (CHC).[8] Single doses of AB68 ranging from 0.25 to 40 mg were administered to 15 subjects and multiple doses of ranging from 10 to 120 mg were administered to 25 subjects. The study drug was administered weekly for 3 weeks, then 3 times a week for the fourth week, and patients were monitored during a subsequent 3-month period.

The investigators report that the drug was well tolerated in all the subjects without moderate or severe adverse effects, and no pattern of drug-induced adverse effect was recorded. Of the 15 subjects who received single doses, 6 presented with a transient 2- to 100-fold reduction in HCV RNA levels immediately after drug administration, but HCV RNA levels returned to baseline within 24 to 48 hours. Also, of the 25 patients in the multiple dose group, 8 presented with at least a 1-log decrease in HCV RNA levels, and the remaining 17 patients showed at least a 0.75-log decrease in HCV

RNA levels from baseline at some point in the course of the study. Again, this study underscores the potential ability of AB68 to safely treat the HCV infection.

Despite these promising findings, XTL Biopharmaceuticals announced in 2003 that AB68 would no longer be investigated in isolation, but in combination with another monoclonal antibody, AB65. The decision to combine the 2 antibodies was based on preclinical studies indicating that combination was more effective against HCV infection. A phase I study of the monoclonal cocktail has been initiated and AB6865 has been granted fast-track designation.[10,19]

As with AB68, AB65 was generated from peripheral blood mononuclear cells that were harvested from a donor with asymptomatic HCV infection. Preclinical studies show that the AB6865 combination can identify different conformational epitopes on E2. In addition, AB6865 can immunoprecipitate HCV particles from infected patients' sera that contain different strains of the virus. AB6865 does not activate complement-dependent or antibody-dependent cytotoxicity, but instead induces phagocytosis of the immune complexes by neutrophils, which implies that the antibodies' mode of viral clearance involves endocytosis. Work with the HCV-Trimera mouse model shows that the AB6865 antibody combination significantly inhibits HCV infection of liver fragments, and also reduces the viral load in HCV-infected animals. Various methods were used to demonstrate the potential of AB6865 against HCV infection.[10,19] Although clinical studies have been initiated, no published data are yet available.

Bavituximab

Bavituximab is a monoclonal antibody with a unique mechanism of action. It is the first in a new class of specifically targeted antiphosphatidylserine (anti-PS) antibodies. These antibodies bind to a specific phospholipid component of cell membranes known as phosphatidylserine.[20] Phosphatidylserine is a lipid molecule normally found in the interior of cellular membranes. However, it becomes exposed on the cell membranes of enveloped viruses and virally infected cells during replication. The internal positioning of phosphatidylserine is maintained by ATP-dependent aminophospholipid translocases.[21] These molecules catalyze aminophospholipid transport from the outside to the inside surface of the plasma membrane. Investigators suggest that phosphatidylserine is present on the external membrane surface of virally infected cells only when the viruses activate host cells to replicate.[21] This causes an increase in intracellular calcium, which in turn leads to phosphatidylserine externalization by activating phosphatidylserine exporters and inhibiting phosphatidylserine import by translocases.

It has been argued that the presence of phosphatidylserine on the outer membranes of viruses enable them to "evade immune recognition," and dampens the body's normal response to infection.[21] Thus by binding cells with exposed phosphatidylserine, bavituximab may help block the immunosuppressive signals from such viruses and allow the body to develop an effective immune response. Bavituximab has 2 major advantages over other antibodies being developed for treatment of HCV and other chronic viral infections. First, because the molecule targeted by the drug is found only on virally infected cells, it should be specific for infected cells and spare healthy ones. Second, because the targeted molecule is a feature of the host cell and not the virus itself, the drug is less likely to lose its effectiveness due to viral mutations. Because bavituximab works by identifying a molecule common to viral infections in general, not just HCV, it is being developed as a potential therapy for other chronic viral infections such as HIV, cytomegalovirus (CMV), influenza, and a host of others.

A preclinical study has tested the notion that phosphatidylserine exposure is common to all viral infections, and whether bavituximab's antiviral activity is effective in all cases of exposed phosphatidylserine.[21] Bavituximab binding was tested in cells infected with influenza A, vesicular stomatitis virus (VSV), and mouse cytomegalovirus (mCMV). In all cases phosphatidylserine exposure was induced, as detected by flow cytometry and fluorescence microscopy. In the same study, bavituximab was reported to effectively cure guinea pigs infected with Pichinde virus. The drug was also reported to be capable of binding with and treating several other viral infections, such as mice infected with lethal mouse cytomegalovirus. Bavituximab is believed to achieve this antiviral activity through direct clearance and antibody-dependent cellular cytotoxicity, and seems to be effective.[21]

A phase I clinical study testing the safety, tolerability, and the pharmacokinetics of bavituximab was reported in 2007 at the 58th Annual Meeting of the American Association for the Study of Liver Diseases (AASLD).[9] Of the total 24 patients enrolled in the study, 15 were male with average age of 49 years, 11 were nonresponders, 8 were relapsers, and 5 were treatment-naive patients. The mean baseline viral load was 5 million copies per milliliter. Fifteen of the 24 patients were infected with HCV genotype 1, 8 had genotype 3, and 1 had genotype 2. The subjects were divided into 4 groups of 6 patients with each group receiving 90-minute intravenous infusions for 2 weeks at 0.3, 1, 3, or 6 mg/kg. The patients were followed for 12 weeks during which vital signs, physical examination, serum bavituximab levels, and HCV RNA levels were measured.

A decline of greater than 0.5 log10 reduction in HCV RNA was reported for 5 of 6 patients receiving 3 mg/kg, suggesting a modest antiviral effect. In addition, no serious adverse effects and no early discontinuations due to drug-related factors were reported. The researchers concluded that twice-weekly intravenous doses of bavituximab at up to 6 mg/kg are safe, well tolerated, and effective. Further studies investigating appropriate dosing schedules and the combination of bavituximab with other drugs were recommended.[9]

Civacir

Civacir is one of a few polyclonal antibodies under investigation for its ability to neutralize HCV infection and thus prevent reinfection of HCV-positive patients who have undergone liver transplantation. Civacir, also known as human hepatitis C immune globulin, is obtained from human plasma enriched with HCV polyclonal antibodies collected from screened donors. The plasma is purified and the antibodies that neutralize HCV are concentrated in a process known as fractionation.[22] A controlled, phase I/II, randomized, open-label, multicenter study was initiated in 2004 to test the tolerability, safety, and pharmacokinetics of this polyclonal antibody.[22]

The study enrolled adults with decompensated chronic HCV who were listed for liver transplantation. A total of 18 patients listed for transplants in 4 different centers were enrolled and randomized into 3 groups: low dose, high dose, and a control group. To ensure similar proportions of randomization, each transplant center was provided with its own randomization sequence. A time-dependent dosing strategy was designed for the study. Each group, with the exception of the control group, received a total of 17 intravenous infusions over the study period in the following sequence: during liver reperfusion, 8 to 12 hours after transplantation, and on post-transplantation days 1, 2, 3, 4, 7, 10, 14, 17, 21, 28, 35, 42, 56, 70, and 98. The patients were then followed for another 12 weeks after the last infusion on day 98. To evaluate the safety and antiviral activity of the drug, blood was collected from the subjects on study days 4 to 7, 10 to 14, 21, 28, 35, 42, 56, 70, 98, 99, 102, 105, 112, 126, and 154, and the total anti-HCV and anti-E2 antibodies antibody levels were measured.[22]

The results showed that the half-life of Civacir was short immediately after liver transplantation, but was gradually prolonged at longer intervals after surgery. No patient developed hepatic fibrosis and serum alanine aminotransferase (ALT) levels normalized in most patients during the study, but no significant reduction in HCV RNA levels was recorded in any dose group. The researchers concluded that the study drug seems to be well tolerated and safe in high and low doses in patients undergoing liver transplantation, but further studies are required to determine whether the drug has beneficial antiviral activity against HCV infection.

PRECLINICAL DEVELOPMENT

Several monoclonal and polyclonal antibodies against HCV are in preclinical stages of investigation. If they are effective in animals, clinical studies will be initiated to assess their safety and pharmacokinetics in humans. The variety of drugs in this stage of development is diverse; this review is limited to antibodies that attack HCV at the receptor level (point of entry) and seem promising as effective therapies or vaccines for HCV.

Membrane receptors on the surface of host cells play an important role in the entry of HCV into the cell, therefore several investigations of receptor protein inhibitors are in preclinical stages. For instance, CD81, Scavenger receptor class BI (SR-BI), tight junction claudin proteins, and other receptors play a mediating role in HCV cell entry,[11] and attempts are being made to inhibit these receptors to protect against HCV infection. However, a potentially more promising endeavor focuses on the development of a vaccine that could provide passive protection against HCV infection. Vanwolleghem and colleagues[17] reported that immunoglobulin G (IgG) from chronically infected patients might be a good candidate for this type of vaccine. In a preclinical study, these investigators injected chimeric mice with immunoglobulin G collected from patients suffering chronic hepatitis C infection. Three days later, the mice were challenged with a 100% infectious dose of the acute phase HCV. The investigators report that in 5 of the 8 challenged mice, passive immunity derived from the injected immunoglobulin-induced sterilizing immunity against HCV infection.[17]

Law and colleagues[7] have taken this research further. They were able to isolate polyclonal antibodies that broadly neutralize several strains of HCV, supporting the notion that vaccines for HCV are indeed attainable. The investigators first isolated 115 clones that showed specific binding to HCV E2 glycoprotein from an antibody antigen-binding fragment (Fab) generated from the blood of a donor with CHC. From these 115 clones, 7 Fabs that could recognize and bind with the 3 antigenic regions of E2 were isolated and converted into full-length immunoglobulins G. The monoclonal antibodies derived from these immunoglobulins were tagged AR1, AR2, and AR3. Whereas the 3 antibodies bind with HCV genotypes 1, E1, and E2, only AR3 showed neutralizing effects.[7]

To test the protective function of the 2 variants of AR3 (AR3A and AR3B), the antibodies were administered intraperitoneally in mice with high levels of human liver chimerism. The mice were later challenged with human HCV-infected serum intravenously. All 4 animals in the control group were infected and the serum viral load was maintained at more than 10,000 RNA copies/ml until the completion of the study. In animals injected with AR3A (n = 5) or AR3B (n = 4), HCV was detected a day after the challenge in 5 (of 9) animals, but was cleared 6 days after the infection. Although increasing levels of HCV RNA were found in some of the animals 2 to 4 weeks after the challenge, some of the animals were still protected at week 6, when the antibody was decreased to less than 10% of the original concentration injected. The investigators conclude that the antibodies indeed protect against HCV infection, although high concentrations may be required for protection. Thus the prospects of developing a vaccine for HCV seem possible.[7]

SUMMARY

As noted throughout this issue, HCV infection constitutes one of the major health burdens facing the world. CHC currently accounts for most of the 5000 annual liver transplants in the United States and records between 10,000 and 12,000 deaths. Unfortunately, the currently approved drug regimens have relatively low efficacy (especially for HCV genotype 1) and a significant side effect profile. Furthermore, reinfection posttransplantation is universal. The need to develop effective preventive and therapeutic drugs for HCV is urgently needed. This goal is a daunting task, given that HCV exists as several distinct strains and is characterized by frequent mutation. Monoclonal and polyclonal antibodies offer strong constituent products for antiviral drugs. In theory, antibodies have the potential to be more effective than other antiviral approaches because they target specific molecular mechanisms of the disease: they can simply intercept viral invaders and prompt the body's immune system to act; they can block the entry of viruses into host cells by targeting host cell receptors; and they can be made to follow viral substances into the host cell and neutralize them. Despite the theoretical opportunities offered by this approach, to date no antibody therapies have been proven to be more than transiently effective in animals or humans.

In addition to the challenges posed by the virus itself, several other factors contribute to these shortcomings, the most notable being the paucity of ongoing research in this area. There are presently only 4 drugs in the clinical stage of development and only a handful in the preclinical stage. These research efforts must be increased and improved if the full potential of monoclonal and polyclonal antibodies is to be maximized in treating and preventing HCV. Monoclonal and polyclonal antibodies to the HCV envelope proteins may present a promising option for effective treatment, alone or in combination with other new anti-HCV regimens.

REFERENCES

1. Theodore SM, Jamal M. Epidemiology of hepatitis C virus (HCV) infection. Int J Med Sci 2006;3(2):41–6.
2. Cholongitas E, Papatheodoridis GV. Review article: novel therapeutic options for chronic hepatitis C. Aliment Pharmacol Ther 2008;27:866–84.
3. Armstrong GL, Wasley A, Simard EP, et al. The prevalence of hepatitis C virus infection in the United States, 1999 through 2002. Ann Intern Med 2006;144:705–14.
4. Borgia G. Specific immunoglobulin against HCV: new perspectives. IDrugs 2004;7(6):570–4.
5. Worman HJ. Current treatment of hepatitis C and its complications. In: The hepatitis C sourcebook. New York: McGraw-Hill; 2002. p. 14, 83–121.
6. Farci P, Alter HJ, Wong DC, et al. Prevention of hepatitis C virus infection in chimpanzees after antibody-mediated in vitro neutralization. Proc Natl Acad Sci U S A 1994;91(16):7792–6.
7. Law M, Maruyama T, Lewis J, et al. Broadly neutralizing antibodies protect against hepatitis C virus quasispecies challenge. Nat Med 2008;14(1):25–9.
8. Galun E, Terrault NA, Eren R, et al. Clinical evaluation (phase I) of a human monoclonal antibody against hepatitis C virus: safety and antiviral activity. J Hepatol 2007;46:37–44.

9. Lawitz EJ, Godofsky EW and Shan JS. Multiple dose safety and pharmacokinetic study of bavituximab in patients with chronic hepatitis C virus (HCV) infection. 58th Annual Meeting of the American Association for the Study of Liver Diseases (AASLD) Boston, MA. Nov 2–6, 2007. Available at: http://www.natap.org/2007/AASLD/AASLD_74.htm. Accessed February 7, 2009.
10. Eren R, Landstein D, Terkieltaub D, et al. Preclinical evaluation of two neutralizing human monoclonal antibodies against hepatitis C virus (HCV): a potential treatment to prevent HCV reinfection in liver transplant patients. J Virol 2006;80(6):2654–64.
11. Stamataki Z, Grove J, Balfe P, et al. Hepatitis C virus entry and neutralization. Clin Liver Dis 2008;12:693–712.
12. Pawlotsky J, Chaveliez S, McHutchison JG. The hepatitis C virus life cycle as a target for new antiviral therapies. Gastroenterology 2007;132:1979–98.
13. Hsu M, Zhang J, Flint M, et al. Hepatitis C virus glycoproteins mediate pH-dependent cell entry of pseudotyped retroviral particles. Proc Natl Acad Sci U S A 2003;100:7271–6.
14. Tscherne DM, Jones CT, Evans MJ, et al. Time and temperature-dependent activation of hepatitis C virus for low-pH-triggered entry. J Virol 2006;80:1734–41.
15. Blanchard E, Belouzard S, Goueslain L, et al. Hepatitis C virus entry depends on clathrin-mediated endocytosis. J Virol 2006;80:6964–72.
16. Reichert JM. Trends in the development and approval of monoclonal antibodies for viral infections. BioDrugs 2007;21(1):1–7.
17. Vanwolleghem T, Bukh J, Meuleman P, et al. Polyclonal immunoglobulins from a chronic hepatitis C virus patient protect human liver–chimeric mice from infection with a homologous hepatitis C virus strain. Hepatology 2008;47(6):1846–55.
18. Schiano TD, Charlton M, Younossi Z, et al. Monoclonal antibody HCV-AbXTL68 in patients undergoing liver transplantation for HCV: results of a phase 2 randomized study. Liver Transpl 2006;12:1381–9.
19. Borgia G. HepeX-C XTL Biopharmaceuticals. IDrugs 2004;5(8):892–8.
20. Bavituximab. Peregrine Pharmaceuticals Inc. Fall Winter 2008. Available at: http://www.peregrineinc.com/images/stories/media/siteFiles/20081121_BavituximabAV.pdf. Accessed February 7, 2009.
21. Soares MM, King SW, Thorpe PE. Targeting inside-out phosphatidylserine as a therapeutic strategy for viral diseases. Nat Med 2008;14(12):1357–62.
22. Davis GL, Nelson DR, Terrault N, et al. A randomized, open-label study to evaluate the safety and pharmacokinetics of human hepatitis C immune globulin (Civacir) in liver transplant recipients. Liver Transpl 2005;11(8):941–9.

Thrombopoietin Agonists for the Treatment of Thrombocytopenia in Liver Disease and Hepatitis C

Geoffrey Dusheiko, MB, BCh, FCP(SA), FRCP, FRCP(Edin)

KEYWORDS

- Thrombopoietin • Thrombocytopenia
- Cirrhosis • Hepatitis C • Interferon treatment
- Thrombopoietin receptor agonists

Thrombocytopenia is a condition of unusually low level of platelets in blood, resulting from an imbalance between the production and destruction of platelets. Thrombocytopenia is associated with several medical disorders including aplastic anemia, myelodysplasia, and idiopathic thrombocytopenic purpura (ITP). Low platelets can occur as a consequence of myelosuppressive or myeloablative chemotherapy or radiotherapy. Thrombocytopenia can also be associated with severe chronic liver disease as a result of several factors that may act in concert. These include the reduced production of the endogenous thrombopoietic growth factor, thrombopoietin (TPO), and the increased sequestration of platelets within the enlarged spleen.[1] In occasional patients infected with the hepatitis C virus (HCV), thrombocytopenia may apparently occur due to the myelosuppressive effects of the virus on the bone marrow.

Platelet production originates from megakaryocyte precursor cells in the bone marrow. Proliferation and differentiation in the megakaryocytic pathway is predominantly controlled by TPO, a cytokine that is primarily synthesized by the liver and constitutively produced. The binding of TPO to the TPO receptor (TPOr) on cells in the megakaryocyte pathway triggers the activation of the cytoplasmic tyrosine kinases Janus kinase 2 (JAK2) and tyrosine kinase 2 (Tyk2), which in turn activate signal transducers and activators of transcription 5 (STAT5) and phosphoinositide-3 (PI-3) kinase, and Ras-mitogen-activated protein kinase (MAPK).[2] Changes in gene expression in

Centre for Hepatology, Royal Free and University College School of Medicine and Royal Free Hospital, Pond Street, Hampstead London, NW3 2QG, UK
E-mail address: g.dusheiko@medsch.ucl.ac.uk

Clin Liver Dis 13 (2009) 487–501
doi:10.1016/j.cld.2009.05.012
liver.theclinics.com

precursor cells promote differentiation along the megakaryocytic lineage and have an antiapoptotic effect, which ultimately leads to platelet development and release.

CLINICAL SIGNIFICANCE OF THROMBOCYTOPENIA

Critical levels of clinically significant thrombocytopenia in ITP and in other conditions, including liver disease, are under debate. Prevention of hemorrhage is the critical issue, however. In emergencies, hemorrhage due to thrombocytopenia is managed by platelet transfusions. There is some evidence that the prevention of bleeding during the treatment of malignant disease may improve outcomes.

THROMBOCYTOPENIA IN CIRRHOSIS

Thrombocytopenia (defined as platelet counts less than 150,000/μL) is a common manifestation seen in patients with chronic liver disease. The condition is frequent in patients with cirrhosis and advanced cirrhosis and is a hallmark of this stage of the disease.[3] Up to 75% of patients with cirrhosis may have thrombocytopenia (defined as platelet counts of less than 150,000/μL). In advanced liver disease and decompensated cirrhosis more severe degrees of thrombocytopenia may occur, and indeed platelet counts correlate with the degree of fibrosis. Thirteen percent of patients with cirrhosis have moderate degrees of thrombocytopenia, defined as platelet concentrations of 50,000/μL to 75,000/μL.[1] Although patients without cirrhosis may have thrombocytopenia occasionally, patients with cirrhosis have a far greater likelihood of thrombocytopenia. Thrombocytopenia per se may not be a major clinical problem in cirrhosis but low platelet counts can increase the bleeding risk with invasive procedures.[1]

Compensatory mechanisms are often operative in liver disease and therefore account for the degree of hemostatic balance that is frequently observed in these patients despite thrombocytopenia and prolongation of the prothrombin time. Indeed thrombin generation in patients with cirrhosis and abnormal standard coagulation tests is similar to that of healthy individuals.[4,5] However, the ability to initiate and maintain interferon (IFN) treatment of patients with hepatitis B and C and low platelet counts may offset treatment adherence and hence outcome. Growth factors are commonly used to increase hemoglobin and neutrophils.[6] There are currently no data to indicate improvement in sustained virological response (SVR) if platelet counts are increased, but the question remains of considerable interest.

The cause of thrombocytopenia in liver disease is apparently multifactorial. The perceived wisdom is that the low platelet counts are due to hypersplenism and splenic platelet sequestration secondary to portal hypertension. However, additional factors can contribute to the development of thrombocytopenia. More recent insights suggest that increased platelet breakdown and to a lesser extent decreased platelet production play a more important role than previously believed. These include reductions in the hepatic production of the hematopoietic growth factor TPO due to a functional decrease in liver tissue.[1,7] Serum TPO levels are significantly lower in thrombocytopenic patients with cirrhosis compared with nonthrombocytopenic and control groups.[4,8,9] In some cases bone marrow suppression associated with chronic hepatitis C infection and antiviral treatment with IFN-based therapy reduces platelet counts.[10] Immune associated platelet clearance due to platelet antibodies including anti-GPIIb/IIIa antibody has been reported in liver disease and in hepatitis C.[9,11–13] These factors may play a synergistic role.

In addition to the reduction in platelet number, other studies suggest the existence of functional platelet defects, perhaps secondary to soluble plasma factors. These defects reflect not only a decrease in aggregation ability but also an activation of the intrinsic inhibitory pathways. Recent data suggest that platelets may also contribute to the liver disease process as, for instance, in viral hepatitis and cholestatic liver disease.[14] Platelets administered in the mouse carbon tetrachloride model may reduce hepatic fibrosis.[15]

Thrombocytopenia is one of the major adverse effects of IFN-α treatment and will often preclude patients from treatment, or necessitate dose reductions or treatment discontinuation in patients with advanced liver disease. Low platelet counts may thus affect response[16] although the effect may reflect other variables in these patients. However, there is little information on how IFN-α inhibits human megakaryopoiesis. It has been demonstrated that IFN-α does not inhibit colony formation of megakaryocytes from human CD34(+) hematopoietic stem cells or endomitosis, but does inhibit cytoplasmic maturation of megakaryocytes and platelet production in vitro. IFN-α suppresses the expression of transcription factors regulating late-stage megakaryopoiesis, such as GATA-1, p45(NF-E2), and MafG. IFN-α also significantly reduces the number of platelets in circulation but not megakaryocytes.[17] Based on ultrastructural studies, IFN-α may inhibit the maturation of demarcation membranes in megakaryocytes.[17]

Thrombocytopenia is a common finding in liver transplant candidates, and complicates their surgery. Transplantation for decompensated cirrhosis may be jeopardized because of the risk of bleeding due to thrombocytopenia, and reduced functional status of platelets that persist after orthotopic liver transplantation. After liver transplantation, platelet counts may further decrease before increasing after the second to third week post transplant due to increased production of liver TPO.[18–20]

TPO: STRUCTURE AND FUNCTION

TPO is a large molecule of 95 kDa (333 amino acids) which was only discovered in 1991 and purified and cloned in 1994.[21] TPO is the primary physiologic regulator of platelet production and is thus the central regulator of megakaryocytopoeisis and a potent stimulator of platelet synthesis. TPO is known to bind the TPO receptor. TPO is also variously termed thrombopoietin, megapoietin, megakaryocyte growth and development factor, or c-mpl ligand. The TPO receptor is found on megakaryocyte precursor cells, megakaryocytes, and platelets, and on stem cells and bone marrow progenitor cells.[21,22]

The receptor-binding domain of TPO, which binds to the c-Mpl receptor, is responsible for the biologic function of the molecule. Each TPO molecule binds 2 TPO receptors. The domain shares a remarkable homology with erythropoietin at the primary sequence level and tertiary structure. TPO is organized into 4 a helices; the crystal structure is known. Production of TPO is regulated by constitutive production and is reduced only in liver disease; no storage form of the protein exists. TPO is cleared by TPO receptors on platelets.[23] If platelet production is reduced, circulating levels of TPO increase as the clearance of TPO decreases.

DRUG TREATMENTS FOR THROMBOCYTOPENIA

The discovery of platelet growth factors provided an anticipated method of abrogating thrombocytopenia. Several first-generation TPOs were tested for their ability to overcome thrombocytopenia. The first-generation recombinant thrombopoietic growth factors and the pegylated moiety, PEG-rHuMGDF, investigated in the mid 1990s and early 2000s, proved effective in increasing platelet count in normal volunteers, in thrombocytopenia due to chemotherapy, and also in a few cases of idiopathic thrombocytopenic purpura (ITP); recombinant human TPO given by subcutaneous injection for chemotherapy-induced thrombocytopenia resulted in a shorter platelet recovery time in lung cancer.[24] Studies in humans showed that platelet count increased in response to the administration of TPO; there was typically a lag time of approximately 5 days, and platelet counts peaked by days 12 to 14 with linear response curves. However, the results of early trials were disappointing.[25] During chemotherapy for lung cancer, nadir platelet counts increased and there was some reduction in the need for platelet transfusions. Treatment of thrombocytopenia inpatients with leukemia did not translate into major clinical benefit; there was some demonstrable benefit for ITP and myelodysplastic syndrome. Unfortunately, the clinical development of these first-generation compounds was stopped after larger safety studies indicated the induction of antibody to recombinant TPO in some recipients.[23] The development of IgG4 antibody to PEG-rHuMGDF that cross-reacted with endogenous TPO neutralized its activity and thereby led to treatment-induced thrombocytopenia.[25]

Pleiotropic cytokines have been shown to have a generally modest effect on thrombocytopenia. In particular, interleukin (IL)-11 has successfully been shown to reduce the incidence of severe thrombocytopenia in patients receiving intensive chemotherapy, and has been approved by the US Food and Drug Administration (FDA) for the treatment of severe thrombocytopenia in patients receiving myelosuppressive therapy. However, side effects are common and particularly limiting in patients with liver disease.[26]

SECOND-GENERATION THROMBOPOIETIC GROWTH FACTORS

Second-generation thrombopoietic growth factors, having no sequence homology with natural TPO, have been developed.[27] These are consequently nonimmunogenic. Several classes have been developed. These include (1) TPO peptide mimetics, (2) TPO nonpeptide mimetics, and (3) TPO antibody mimetics.[21,22,28]

These second-generation compounds have different modes of activation on the TPO receptor; the first 2 have been most extensively studied in the clinic.[22] The 2 most studied agents are romiplostim, a peptibody, and eltrombopag, a nonpeptide, orally active small molecule. In open-label and placebo-controlled trials both agents predictably increase platelet counts in normal volunteers and in patients with ITP.

Romiplostin (Nplate, Amgen)

Romiplostin was identified in 1997.[29] The initial name of romiplostin was Amgen Megakaryopoiesis Protein-2 (AMP-2), and AMG 531. Romiplostin is a 60-kDa structure constituted by 4 TPO mimetic peptides attached by glycine bridges to a novel IgG heavy-chain Fc region, a recombinant protein defined as a peptibody:[30] L-methionyl [human immunoglobulin heavy constant gamma 1-(227 C-terminal residues)-peptide (Fc fragment)]. The compound is a recombinant fusion protein which contains 2 identical single-chain subunits. Romiplostin activates the TPO receptor by binding to the distal receptor domain. Dimerization increases the specific activity by allowing binding to 2 TPO receptors. The initial poor activity of the compound was improved by molecular changes that stabilized the peptide after incorporation into immunoglobulin carrier molecules. The 14-amino-acid peptide bears no sequence homology with endogenous TPO, but activates the TPO receptor.

The circulatory half-life of romiplostin is 120 to 160 hours; the peptide is cleared by the reticuloendothelial system. For therapeutic use, romiplostin is constituted as a lyophilized powder for reconstitution with water and injected subcutaneously at doses of 1 to 10 μg/kg weekly.[31,32] Romiplostin was approved in 2008 by the FDA for the treatment of chronic ITP in patients who showed an insufficient response to first-line therapies including corticosteroids, immunoglobulins, or splenectomy.

Eltrombopag

Eltrombopag (Promacta/Revolade; GlaxoSmithKline) was formerly known as SB497115. The compound was identified by screening libraries designed to identify structures that could activate the TPO receptor. Eltrombopag is a member of the biarylhydrazone class of compounds, with an empirical formula of $C_{25}H_{22}N_4O_4$ and a molecular weight of 442.47 (**Fig. 1**).[33] Eltrombopag is a small molecule, nonpeptide, mimetic agonist of the thrombopoietin receptor (TPOr). Eltrombopag binds to the transmembrane region; it has been suggested that it activates the receptor by association with metal ions (ie, Zn^{2+}) and specific amino acids within the transmembrane and juxtamembrane domains of the TPOr (**Figs. 2** and **3**). The compound thus activates signaling transducers and activators of transcription (STAT) and mitogen-activated protein kinase signal transduction pathways. In a variety of different assays, eltrombopag showed no activity in cells expressing receptors for other hematopoietic growth factors that are activated by STAT, including erythropoietin, granulocyte-colony stimulating factor (G-CSF), and interferon. Eltrombopag activates only human and chimpanzee STAT pathways: histidine 499 in the TPO receptor transmembrane region is necessary for the reactivity to the thrombopoietin mimetics and confers this species specificity.[34] The activity of eltrombopag is dependent on the expression of TPOr. Eltrombopag and TPO do not bind to the same site on the TPOr, which prevents competitive binding and allows eltrombopag and TPO to have additive cell signaling effects.

Eltrombopag interacts specifically with the TPOr without competing with TPO, thereby activating intracellular signal transduction pathways additively with endogenous TPO, leading to the increased proliferation and differentiation of human bone marrow progenitor cells into megakaryocytes and ultimately, increased platelet production.[35] The net result is the facilitation of megakaryocyte differentiation into platelets. Assessment of megakaryocyte maturation can be determined by measuring the appearance of the megakaryocyte-specific marker glycoprotein CD41 on human

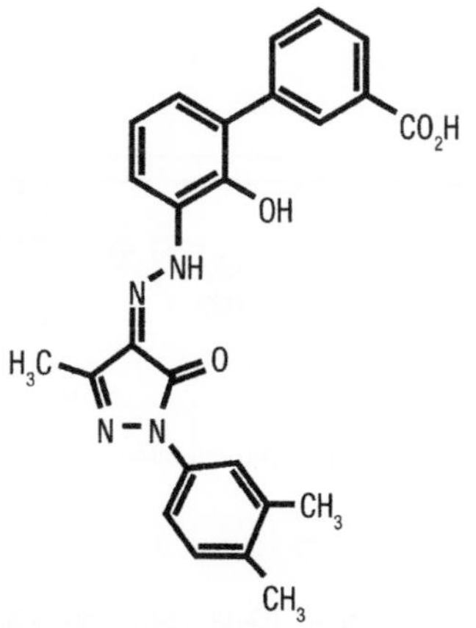

Fig. 1. Structure of eltrombopag.

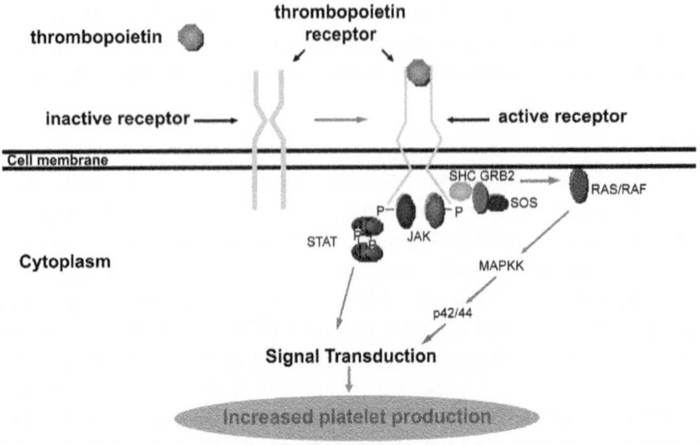

Fig. 2. Mechanism of action of thrombopoietin. (*Data from* Kaushansky K. Lineage-specific hematopoietic growth factors. N Engl J Med 2006;354:2034–45.)

CD34+ cells obtained from human bone marrow samples. Functional thrombopoietic activity has been demonstrated by proliferation and differentiation of primary human CD34+ bone cells into CD41+ megakaryocytes. In addition to a proliferative effect on cells of the megakaryocytic lineage, eltrombopag also induces differentiation of hematopoietic stem cells into committed megakaryocyte progenitor cells.

Oral administration of 10 mg/kg eltrombopag per day to chimpanzees was shown to increase platelet counts after 5 days of administration, which is similar to the kinetics of rhTPO.[33,35–38] Eltrombopag EC_{50} values are in the range of 30 to 300 nM. Oral administration of eltrombopag leads to a steady-state minimal concentration of greater than 225 ng/mL and an area under the curve (AUC) of 30 ng h/mL,[35] which were assessed as minimally effective pharmacokinetic parameters for human studies.

The compound is orally bioavailable, and is given orally once a day as 25-, 50-, or 75-mg tablets. Absorption is affected by food and antacids. A single dose has no

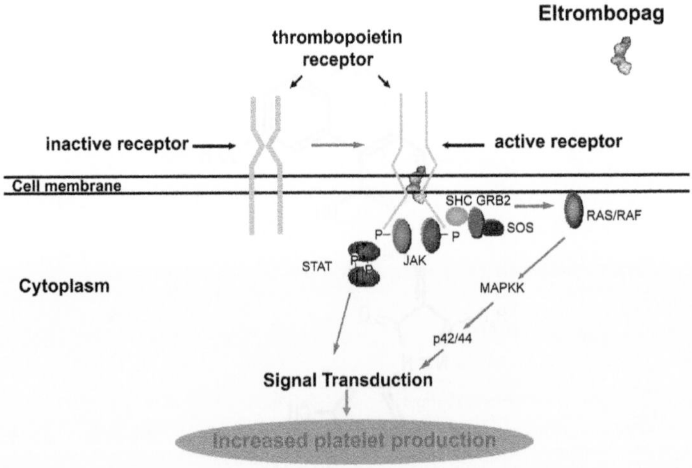

Fig. 3. Mechanism of action ofeltrombopag. (*Data from* Braun BS, Gavin J, Tuveson DA, et al. In vitro analysis of myeloid proliferation caused by oncogenic KRAS. Blood 2004;104(11);795a–7a.)

effect on platelets, but continuous dosing for 10 days results in peak platelet counts at day 16 in healthy volunteers.[33,37,39] When given at doses of 50 to 75 mg/day orally, eltrombopag induces a platelet increase that peaks between 10 and 14 days. Because the compound is a small molecule thrombopoietin mimetic, it is less likely to be immunogenic. Eltrombopag is now approved for the treatment of ITP in the United States.

OTHER COMPOUNDS

Several other analogues are in further pharmaceutical development. Most are small 400- to 900-Da chemical structures. Other agonists based on the benzo[*a*]carbazole ring system[40,41] have been developed. Butyzamide is an orally bioavailable human Mpl activator, and seems to have potential for clinical development as a therapeutic agent for patients with thrombocytopenia.[42] Strategies are in progress to address the chemical instability of the ethylene bridge while retaining or improving functional potency in the agonism of the TPO receptor.

Several of these nonpeptide thrombopoietin-mimetic agonists elicit signal transduction responses comparable with recombinant human TPO, and activate the TPO-dependent cell line Ba/F3-huMPL.[43] AKR-501 (YM477) is an orally active thrombopoietin (TPO) receptor agonist that mimics the biologic effect of TPO in vitro and in vivo. AKR-501 in combination with TPO has an additive effect on megakaryocytopoiesis and TPO mimetic activities.[44,45] RWJ-800088 is a novel thrombopoietin mimetic peptide that seems to increase burst-forming units-erythroid and colony-forming unit counts, suggesting some effects on progenitor lineages.[46]

CLINICAL USE OF TPO AGONISTS

Studies in chemotherapy-induced thrombocytopenia, HCV-related thrombocytopenia, and myelodysplastic syndromes have been completed. Advanced phase I and II studies have been completed in ITP and hepatitis C (**Fig. 4**).

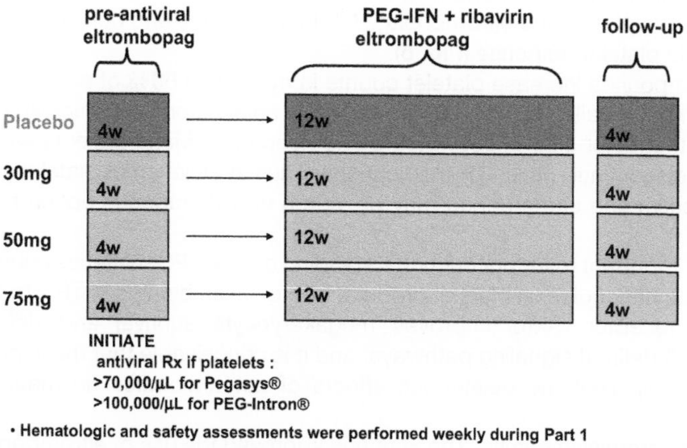

Fig. 4. HCV phase 2 study with eltrombopag: protocol. (*Data from* McHutchison JG, Dusheiko G, Shiffman ML, et al. Eltrombopag for thrombocytopenia in patients with cirrhosis associated with hepatitis C. N Engl J Medicine 2007;357:2227–36.)

STUDIES IN ITP

ITP affects more than 50,000 people in the United States. The pathophysiology is still incompletely understood. The mechanism of idiopathic (autoimmune) thrombocytopenic purpura (ITP) has historically been attributed to platelet autoantibody production and the resultant platelet destruction in the spleen.[47] More recent evidence suggests a multifactorial pathogenesis. A complex picture of the immune processes involved in autoimmunity has emerged over the last decade with the identification and characterization of immunoregulatory elements (receptors, cytokines, and other signaling molecules) and cell trafficking patterns.[47] Autoantibodies against megakaryocyte surface glycoproteins inhibit megakaryocyte growth and development. It has been shown that T cells are activated on recognition of platelet-specific antigens, presented on antigen-presenting cells. Activated T cells, in turn, induce antigen-specific expansion of B cells producing autoantibodies with specificity for GPIIb-IIIa or GPIb-V-IX expressed on platelets and megakaryocytes.[47] Platelets bound by autoantibody are targeted for removal by low-affinity Fc receptors predominantly expressed on splenic macrophages. Autoantibodies also target megakaryocytes by reducing their capacity to produce nascent platelets.[48] TPO levels are usually normal.[30,47,49–51]

Oral corticosteroids are the first line of treatment for ITP, followed by intravenous immune, anti-D immunoglobulin, intravenous methylprednisolone, and splenectomy to treat refractory cases. Other immunosuppressant medications are also used. The mainstay of immunosuppressive treatment is to inhibit autoantibody production by B cells and to thereby reduce clearance of platelets. However, a proportion of patients fail to respond. It has been noted that megakaryocytes are structurally abnormal.[51]

As the disease is characterized by platelet destruction and is also mediated by inappropriately low platelet production; the failure of the bone marrow to maximally increase platelet production seems to play an important role in the thrombocytopenia of ITP and provides a rationale for the use of TPO mimetics to increase platelet production.

Treatment strategies targeting the TPOr to increase platelet production are a promising new approach to the management of ITP. Based on the rationale that the TPOr agonists eltrombopag and romiplostim bind and activate the TPO-R c-Mpl, enhancing platelet production, phase I and II randomized controlled studies have been undertaken with romiplostin and eltrombopag.[37,50] In general the end point of these studies was durable platelet response (**Fig. 5**).

Both compounds increase platelet counts in more than 80% of patients, including patients who had failed first-line treatments and splenectomy. Romiplostim was well tolerated, the major side effect noted being headache. Many patients were able to reduce or discontinue other ITP medications. Thus stimulation of platelet production by romiplostim and eltrombopag may provide a new therapeutic option for patients with ITP.[28,52]

It will be important to further our understanding of how TPO mimetics counteract the effect of autoantibodies on platelet production. However, binding of TPO to the megakaryocyte receptor c-Mpl improves megakaryocyte survival and differentiation through well-defined signaling pathways, and it is conceivable that these pro-survival processes help limit the deleterious effects of autoantibodies on megakaryocyte platelets.[53]

These are promising results. The FDA has approved the use of eltrombopag for the treatment of ITP with an insufficient response to steroids, immunoglobulin, and splenectomy.[27,51] Romiplostin has also been approved for adult patients with ITP.

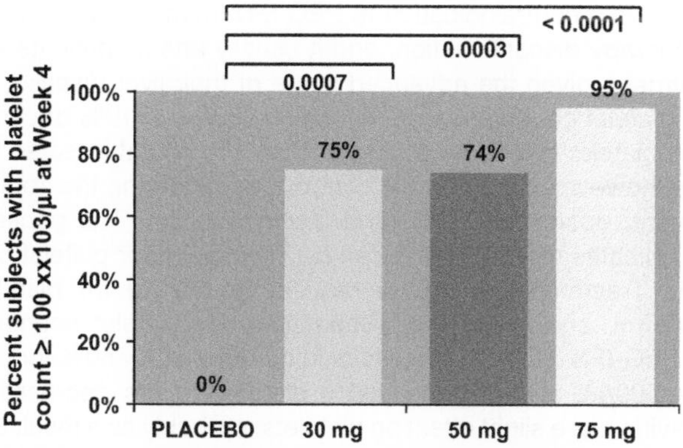

Fig. 5. Primary end point: platelet counts of greater than 100,000µL at week 4. (*Data from* McHutchison JG, Dusheiko G, Shiffman ML et al. Eltrombopag for thrombocytopenia in patients with cirrhosis associated with hepatitis C. N Engl J Medicine 2007;357:2227–36.)

However, the disease and its management remain a challenge. The optimal management of ITP is still unsettled and the use of thrombopoietin agonists for ITP may be restricted to refractory patients. However, given the risks of splenectomy and the understandable reluctance of patients to undergo splenectomy, effective and safe treatments that increase platelet numbers in refractory patients will be a major advance. The response observed to these agents is maintained during treatment, but is almost invariably lost even after several months of successful administration, so that the safety of chronic administration will prove important (**Fig. 6**).

TREATMENT OF THROMBOCYTOPENIA IN HEPATITIS C

Thrombocytopenia observed in patients with hepatitis C is usually encountered in advanced cirrhosis, and is frequently a hallmark of the stage of the disease. Antiviral therapy in thrombocytopenic patients with HCV is a factor in reducing candidacy for current treatment and limiting response to pegylated (PEG)-IFN treatment. Severe

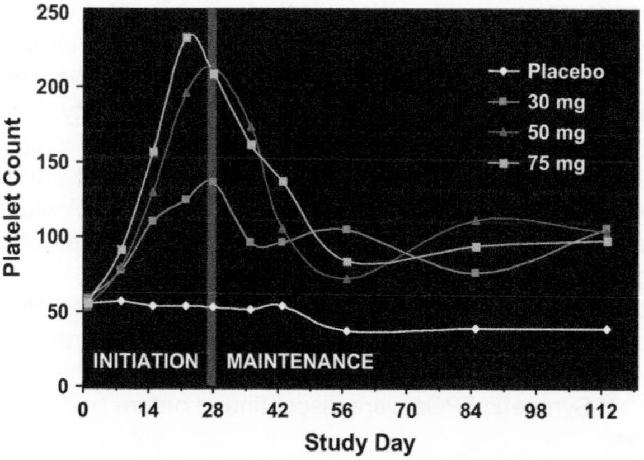

Fig. 6. Dose response curve; median platelet counts with eltrombopag. (*Data from* McHutchison JG, Dusheiko G, Shiffman ML, et al. Eltrombopag for thrombocytopenia in patients with cirrhosis associated with hepatitis C. N Engl J Medicine 2007;357:2227–36.)

thrombocytopenia is a contraindication to PEG-IFN therapy and a cause for dosage reduction and therapy discontinuation, and it usually affects patients who are more in need of treatment, given the advanced stage of their liver disease. Heathcote et al showed that platelet counts fell to less than 50,000/μL in 19% of cirrhotic patients (whose baseline platelet counts were greater than 150,000/μL) treated with PEG-IFN α-2a.[54] There is, however, considerable controversy regarding the appropriate cutoff allowing treatment, dose reductions, and discontinuation. The package insert for PEG-IFN α-2a indicates that treatment can be maintained for platelet counts greater than 50,000/μL. Treatment should be reduced to 90 μg for platelet counts of less than 50,000/mL and should be discontinued for platelet counts of less than 25,000/μL. For PEG-IFN α-2b, the dose should be reduced by 50% for platelet counts of less than 80,000/μL and discontinued if platelet counts decrease to less than 50,000/μL. Ribavirin has a slight effect on platelets, probably as a result of the stimulus of hemolysis, but the effect is modest. In practice, experienced physicians will tailor treatment differently to improve adherence, but great caution and responsibility must be exercised when platelet counts decrease to less than 50,000/μL, and the risks and benefits of treatment require careful weighting. Although practice varies, patients with low platelet counts require more frequent monitoring.

Current treatment of thrombocytopenia in cirrhosis is unsatisfactory. Few options are available. These include platelet transfusions, splenic artery embolism, splenectomy, and transjugular intrahepatic portal systemic shunt (TIPS). When to use such measures remains controversial and practice varies. It seems that spontaneous hemorrhage is rare in uncomplicated cirrhosis with platelet counts of greater than 20,000/μL. Below this level, higher platelet counts are required for medical procedures and interventions. Platelet transfusions are required to provide hemostasis, and procedures with a higher risk of bleeding, surgery, or investigational procedures such as percutaneous liver biopsy are not performed if platelet counts are less than 80,000/μL. However, although transfusions raise platelet counts, the infused platelets are quickly sequestered and the effect is transient and not without complication, and with significant cost. Transjugular liver biopsy can be performed at platelet counts greater than 50,000/μL.[11,18–20] In some studies, large volume paracentesis carries a risk of bleeding at platelet counts of less than 50,000/μL; however, others have shown no association between bleeding complications and platelet count.[9] Hayashi et al[55] investigated whether open splenectomy might improve platelet count and therefore allow PEG-IFN therapy in patients with cirrhosis and HCV infection. In a small series of mainly compensated, thrombocytopenic patients with cirrhosis, open splenectomy led to a significant improvement in platelet count after 221±151 days without detrimental modification of liver function and significant morbidity. This improvement allowed PEG-IFN therapy in 6 out of the 7 patients; a sustained virological response was obtained in 2 patients. However, splenectomy is often ill advised in patients with cirrhosis, who may be candidates for subsequent liver transplantation. Transcatheter arterial partial splenic embolization has been assessed as an alternative by several investigators.[56–62]

Erythropoietin is able to increase platelet count and reverse PEG-IFN-induced thrombocytopenia, and may indeed increase platelet counts. Interleukin-11 proved to be able to increase platelet count in patients with cirrhosis at the cost of significant side effects.[19,26,63] Synthetic TPOs were discontinued before being tested in patients with liver disease.

Eltrombopag has recently been tested in a phase 2 trial. A dose response was demonstrated that was associated with significant increases in platelet counts in a randomized, blinded, controlled clinical trial. Eltrombopag administered to patients with platelets less than 70 × $10^9/\mu L$ for 4 weeks before and during a 12-week course of PEG interferon and ribavirin led to the initiation of therapy in 71% to 91% of treated patients, but only 22% of placebo recipients. Thirty-six percent, 53%, and 65% of patients receiving 30 mg, 50 mg, or 75 mg, respectively, daily compared with 6% in the placebo arm were able to remain on antiviral treatment during the 12-week period of study. Seventy-five milligrams daily given for 4 weeks led to a median platelet count increase from 55,000/μL to 209,000/μL. All treated subjects reached platelet counts of greater than 100,000/μL, but none of the patients receiving placebo increased their platelet count to greater than 100,000/μL. Phase 3 studies are currently in progress to determine whether initiating and maintaining antiviral therapy with eltrombopag will result in increased SVR.[39]

Thrombocytopenia is common during cancer chemotherapy. Small preliminary studies for thrombocytopenia in myelodysplastic syndromes and during chemotherapy are in progress. It is not yet established whether these potent agents will demonstrate clinical effectiveness in these patients and will alter the outlook for the disease.

SAFETY OF SECOND-GENERATION AGENTS

Only short-term exposure studies have been done: 156 weeks for romiplostin and 151 days for eltrombopag. Long-term studies are required. Mild headache has been the most common complaint with these agents. Long-term use will be required to rule out the potential increased risk of new platelet formation and a possible prothrombotic state on thrombosis, increased bone marrow reticulin, rebound worsening of thrombocytopenia, and increased blast formation. To date no increase in thrombosis has been observed. Thromboembolic complications remain a theoretical possibility but have not been observed to be more frequent than placebo. Rebound thrombocytopenia due to increased clearance of endogenous TPO could occur. Increased bone marrow reticulin (which is reversible) has been reported in ITP studies (romiplostin), but to date there is no evidence of a progressive myeloproliferative disorder.[52] Increased reticulin has been reported with TPO. rhTPO may be able to augment the expressions of fibronectin, laminin, and collagen type IV of stromal cells. Preclinical studies have shown an increase in reversible marrow fibrosis.[64,65] The risk of hepatotoxicity with eltrombopag is being closely monitored. It will thus be necessary to institute careful long-term follow-up studies in treated patients.

SUMMARY: THROMBOPOIETIN AGONISTS IN LIVER DISEASE

In the absence of prospective, controlled studies, there is consensus that bleeding risks are significantly greater in patients with liver disease with platelet counts of less than 20,000/μL, and therefore prophylactic treatment of invasive diagnostic and therapeutic procedures is indicated for these patients; for those with platelet counts that are higher, but still less than 50,000/μ, treatment is also indicated if accompanied by substantial mucous membrane bleeding.

The most common coagulation disturbances occurring in liver disease include thrombocytopenia and impaired humoral coagulation. In general the goal of therapy for bleeding is not to achieve complete correction of laboratory value abnormalities but to gain hemostasis. Severe hemorrhage such as variceal bleeding is a medical emergency; thrombocytopenia can impact the emergency and routine care of patients with chronic liver disease. Thrombocytopenia can potentially lead to the postponing of or interference with diagnostic and therapeutic procedures including liver biopsy, antiviral therapy, and medically indicated or elective surgery.[1]

Therapy with vitamin K may be a useful option in patients with increased prothrombin time due to vitamin K deficiency. Infusion of fresh frozen plasma is often effective in liver disease before invasive procedures or surgery, as such patients frequently require transient correction in their prothrombin time. Transfusions of platelets are appropriate for patients with thrombocytopenia (platelet count < 50,000/μL) associated with active bleeding or before invasive procedures in which a short-term platelet count increase is required. A trial with desmopressin may be considered before invasive procedures in patients with liver disease and with refractory and prolonged bleeding time. Recombinant activated factor VIIa administration is suggested for patients with significantly prolonged prothrombin time and contraindications to fresh frozen plasma therapy; however, this is expensive. Interleukin-11 is currently an investigational agent for patients with thrombocytopenia of chronic liver disease.[8]

The development of targeted TPOr agonists has implications for improving therapy for patients with cirrhosis associated with low platelet counts. Data have emerged supporting the role of inadequate platelet production in these patients, and eltrombopag has been successful in boosting platelet counts in patients with cirrhosis due to hepatitis C. These agents are not a substitute for emergency platelet transfusions; there is a time lag for these effects, which could limit the use of these in emergencies but could facilitate elective procedures. These agents are also not curative, and their long-term use has not been studied. Most patients with cirrhosis can tolerate low platelet counts without the need for treatment.

In conclusion, agents that directly stimulate platelet production, such as the second-generation TPOr receptor-binding agents, have shown promise in clinical trials of ITP patients as well as in hepatitis C virus-infected individuals with thrombocytopenia.[66] These agents may provide an important adjunctive treatment option in the future, particularly if response rates to treatment of hepatitis C can be improved by increasing adherence to treatment. The criteria for treatment, and the best strategies remain to be determined.[38,67,68] The cost benefit and cost effectiveness of these adjuncts also require evaluation. The safety of such agents in patients with liver disease and older patients with cirrhosis, vascular disease, and the risk of portal vein thrombosis will require careful assessment.

ACKNOWLEDGMENTS

We are grateful to Dr Julian Jenkins, GSK, for **Figs. 2** to **6**.

REFERENCES

1. Afdhal N, McHutchison J, Brown R, et al. Thrombocytopenia associated with chronic liver disease. J Hepatol 2008;48(6):1000–7.
2. Arnold DM, Kelton JG. Current options for the treatment of idiopathic thrombocytopenic purpura. Semin Hematol 2007;44(4 Suppl 5):S12–23.
3. Poordad F. Review article: thrombocytopenia in chronic liver disease. Aliment Pharmacol Ther 2007;26(Suppl 1):5–11.
4. Caldwell SH, Hoffman M, Lisman T, et al. Coagulation disorders and hemostasis in liver disease: pathophysiology and critical assessment of current management. Hepatology 2006;44(4):1039–46.
5. Tripodi A, Primignani M, Chantarangkul V, et al. Thrombin generation in patients with cirrhosis: the role of platelets. Hepatology 2006;1944:440–5.
6. Tillmann HL, Patel K, McHutchison JG. Role of growth factors and thrombopoietic agents in the treatment of chronic hepatitis C. Curr Gastroenterol Rep 2009;11(1): 5–14.

7. Rajan SK, Espina BM, Liebman HA. Hepatitis C virus-related thrombocytopenia: clinical and laboratory characteristics compared with chronic immune thrombocytopenic purpura. Br J Haematol 2005;129(6):818–24.
8. Blonski W, Siropaides T, Reddy KR. Coagulopathy in liver disease. Curr Treat Options Gastroenterol 2007;10(6):464–73.
9. Giannini EG. Review article: thrombocytopenia in chronic liver disease and pharmacologic treatment options. Aliment Pharmacol Ther 2006;23(8):1055–65.
10. Eissa LA, Gad LS, Rabie AM, et al. Thrombopoietin level in patients with chronic liver diseases. Ann Hepatol 2008;7(3):235–44.
11. Giannini EG, Savarino V. Thrombocytopenia in liver disease. Curr Opin Hematol 2008;15(5):473–80.
12. Pereira J, Accatino L, Alfaro J, et al. Platelet autoantibodies in patients with chronic liver disease. Am J Hematol 1995;50(3):173–8.
13. Pockros PJ, Duchini A, McMillan R, et al. Immune thrombocytopenic purpura in patients with chronic hepatitis C virus infection. Am J Gastroenterol 2002;97(8): 2040–5.
14. Witters P, Freson K, Verslype C, et al. Review article: blood platelet number and function in chronic liver disease and cirrhosis. Aliment Pharmacol Ther 2008; 27(11):1017–29.
15. Watanabe M, Murata S, Hashimoto I, et al. Platelets contribute to the reduction of liver fibrosis in mice. J Gastroenterol Hepatol 2008.
16. Everson GT, Hoefs JC, Seeff LB, et al. Impact of disease severity on outcome of antiviral therapy for chronic hepatitis C: lessons from the HALT-C trial. Hepatology 2006;44(6):1675–84.
17. Yamane A, Nakamura T, Suzuki H, et al. Interferon-alpha 2b-induced thrombocytopenia is caused by inhibition of platelet production but not proliferation and endomitosis in human megakaryocytes. Blood 2008;112(3):542–50.
18. Martin TG III, Somberg KA, Meng YG, et al. Thrombopoietin levels in patients with cirrhosis before and after orthotopic liver transplantation. Ann Intern Med 1997; 127(4):285–8.
19. Peck-Radosavljevic M. Thrombocytopenia in liver disease. Can J Gastroenterol 2000;14(Suppl D):60D–6D.
20. Peck-Radosavljevic M, Wichlas M, Zacherl J, et al. Thrombopoietin induces rapid resolution of thrombocytopenia after orthotopic liver transplantation through increased platelet production. Blood 2000;95(3):795–801.
21. Kuter DJ. Thrombopoietin and thrombopoietin mimetics in the treatment of thrombocytopenia. Annu Rev Public Health 2008.
22. Kuter DJ. New drugs for familiar therapeutic targets: thrombopoietin receptor agonists and immune thrombocytopenic purpura. Eur J Haematol Suppl 2008; 69:9–18.
23. Basser R. Clinical biology and potential use of thrombopoietin. Can J Gastroenterol 2000;14(Suppl D):73D–8D.
24. Xu YH, Chen ZW, Ye XY, et al. [Evaluation of recombinant human thrombopoietin in the treatment of chemotherapy-induced thrombocytopenia in lung cancer patients.]. Zhonghua Zhong Liu Za Zhi 2008;30(9):716–9.
25. Basser R. The impact of thrombopoietin on clinical practice. Curr Pharm Des 2002;8(5):369–77.
26. Fontana V, Dudkiewicz P, Jy W, et al. Interleukin-11 for treatment of hepatitis C-associated ITP. Acta Haematol 2008;119(2):126–32.
27. Rodeghiero F, Ruggeri M. Chronic immune thrombocytopenic purpura. New agents. Hamostaseologie 2009;29(1):76–9.

28. Kuter DJ, Bussel JB, Lyons RM, et al. Efficacy of romiplostim in patients with chronic immune thrombocytopenic purpura: a double-blind randomised controlled trial. Lancet 2008;371(9610):395–403.
29. Cwirla SE, Balasubramanian P, Duffin DJ, et al. Peptide agonist of the thrombopoietin receptor as potent as the natural cytokine. Science 1997;276(5319):1696–9.
30. Stasi R, Evangelista ML, Amadori S. Novel thrombopoietic agents: a review of their use in idiopathic thrombocytopenic purpura. Drugs 2008;68(7):901–12.
31. Wang B, Nichol JL, Sullivan JT. Pharmacodynamics and pharmacokinetics of AMG 531, a novel thrombopoietin receptor ligand. Clin Pharmacol Ther 2004; 76(6):628–38.
32. Zhao YQ, Wang QY, Zhai M, et al. [A multi-center clinical trial of recombinant human thrombopoietin in chronic refractory idiopathic thrombocytopenic purpura]. Zhonghua Nei Ke Za Zhi 2004;43(8):608–10.
33. Jenkins JM, Williams D, Deng Y, et al. Phase 1 clinical study of eltrombopag, an oral, nonpeptide thrombopoietin receptor agonist. Blood 2007;109(11):4739–41.
34. Yamane N, Tanaka Y, Ohyabu N, et al. Characterization of novel non-peptide thrombopoietin mimetics, their species specificity and the activation mechanism of the thrombopoietin receptor. Eur J Pharmacol 2008;586(1–3):44–51.
35. Erickson-Miller CL, Delorme E, Tian SS, et al. Preclinical activity of eltrombopag (SB-497115), an oral, non-peptide thrombopoietin receptor agonist. Stem Cells 2008.
36. Molecule of the month. Eltrombopag. Drug News Perspect 2008;21(6):344.
37. Bussel JB, Cheng G, Saleh MN, et al. Eltrombopag for the treatment of chronic idiopathic thrombocytopenic purpura. N Engl J Med 2007;357(22):2237–47.
38. Lawson A. Eltrombopag in thrombocytopenia. N Engl J Med 2008;358(10): 1072–3.
39. McHutchison JG, Dusheiko G, Shiffman ML, et al. Eltrombopag for thrombocytopenia in patients with cirrhosis associated with hepatitis C. N Engl J Med 2007; 357(22):2227–36.
40. Alper PB, Marsilje TH, Mutnick D, et al. Discovery and biological evaluation of benzo[a]carbazole-based small molecule agonists of the thrombopoietin (Tpo) receptor. Bioorg Med Chem Lett 2008;18(19):5255–8.
41. Marsilje TH, Alper PB, Lu W, et al. Optimization of small molecule agonists of the thrombopoietin (Tpo) receptor derived from a benzo[a]carbazole hit scaffold. Bioorg Med Chem Lett 2008;18(19):5259–62.
42. Nogami W, Yoshida H, Koizumi K, et al. The effect of a novel, small non-peptidyl molecule butyzamide on human thrombopoietin receptor and megakaryopoiesis. Haematologica 2008;93(10):1495–504.
43. Yamane N, Takahashi K, Tanaka Y, et al. Discovery of novel non-peptide thrombopoietin mimetic compounds that induce megakaryocytopoiesis. Biosci Rep 2008; 28(5):275–85.
44. Fukushima-Shintani M, Suzuki K, Iwatsuki Y, et al. AKR-501 (YM477) in combination with thrombopoietin enhances human megakaryocytopoiesis. Exp Hematol 2008;36(10):1337–42.
45. Nakamura T. [Elaboration of a novel small molecule, NIP-004, with thrombopoietin mimetic activities]. Rinsho Ketsueki 2008;49(4):257–62.
46. Liem-Moolenaar M, Cerneus D, Molloy C, et al. Pharmacodynamics and pharmacokinetics of the novel thrombopoietin mimetic peptide RWJ-800088 in humans. Clin Pharmacol Ther 2008.
47. Gernsheimer T. Chronic idiopathic thrombocytopenic purpura: mechanisms of pathogenesis. Oncologist 2009.

48. Wei A, Jackson SP. Boosting platelet production. Nat Med 2008;14(9):917–8.
49. Newland A. Thrombopoietin mimetic agents in the management of immune thrombocytopenic purpura. Semin Hematol 2007;44(4 Suppl 5):S35–45.
50. Pruemer J. Epidemiology, pathophysiology, and initial management of chronic immune thrombocytopenic purpura. Am J Health Syst Pharm 2009;66(2 Suppl 2):S4–10.
51. Psaila B, Bussel JB. Refractory immune thrombocytopenic purpura: current strategies for investigation and management. Br J Haematol 2008;143(1):16–26.
52. Schwartz RS. Immune thrombocytopenic purpura—from agony to agonist. N Engl J Med 2007;357(22):2299–301.
53. Gurney AL, Carver-Moore K, de Sauvage FJ, et al. Thrombocytopenia in c-mpl-deficient mice. Science 1994;265(5177):1445–7.
54. Heathcote EJ, Shiffman ML, Cooksley WG, et al. Peginterferon alfa-2a in patients with chronic hepatitis C and cirrhosis. N Engl J Med 2000;343(23):1673–80.
55. Hayashi PH, Mehia C, Joachim RH, et al. Splenectomy for thrombocytopenia in patients with hepatitis C cirrhosis. J Clin Gastroenterol 2006;40(8):740–4.
56. Annicchiarico BE, Siciliano M, Di SC, et al. Proximal splenic artery embolization allows pegylated interferon and ribavirin combination therapy in chronic hepatitis C virus-infected patients with severe cytopenia. Eur J Gastroenterol Hepatol 2006;18(1):119–21.
57. Barcena R, Gil-Grande L, Moreno J, et al. Partial splenic embolization for the treatment of hypersplenism in liver transplanted patients with hepatitis C virus recurrence before peg-interferon plus ribavirin. Transplantation 2005;79(11):1634–5.
58. Kato M, Shimohashi N, Ouchi J, et al. Partial splenic embolization facilitates completion of interferon therapy in patients with chronic HCV infection and hypersplenism. J Gastroenterol 2005;40(11):1076–7.
59. Moreno A, Barcena R, Blazquez J, et al. Partial splenic embolization for the treatment of hypersplenism in cirrhotic HIV/HCV patients prior to pegylated interferon and ribavirin. Antivir Ther 2004;9(6):1027–30.
60. Palsson B, Verbaan H. Partial splenic embolization as pretreatment for antiviral therapy in hepatitis C virus infection. Eur J Gastroenterol Hepatol 2005;17(11):1153–5.
61. Sohara N, Takagi H, Kakizaki S, et al. The use of partial splenic artery embolization made it possible to administer interferon and ribavirin therapy in a liver transplant patient with fibrosing cholestatic hepatitis C complicated with thrombocytopenia. Transpl Int 2006;19(3):255–7.
62. Unzurrunzaga A, Martinez E, Miguelez JL, et al. Partial splenic embolization as a treatment for hypersplenism in HIV/hepatitis C virus-co-infected patients. AIDS 2007;21(7):885–7.
63. Afdhal NH, McHutchison JG. Review article: pharmacological approaches for the treatment of thrombocytopenia in patients with chronic liver disease and hepatitis C infection. Aliment Pharmacol Ther 2007;26(Suppl 1):29–39.
64. Ceresa IF, Noris P, Ambaglio C, et al. Thrombopoietin is not uniquely responsible for thrombocytosis in inflammatory disorders. Platelets 2007;18(8):579–82.
65. Kaushansky K. Historical review: megakaryopoiesis and thrombopoiesis. Blood 2008;111(3):981–6.
66. Newland A. Emerging strategies to treat chronic immune thrombocytopenic purpura. Eur J Haematol Suppl 2008;69:27–33.
67. Rodeghiero F. First-line therapies for immune thrombocytopenic purpura: re-evaluating the need to treat. Eur J Haematol Suppl 2008;69:19–26.
68. Zimmer J, Hentges F, Andres E. Eltrombopag in thrombocytopenia. N Engl J Med 2008;358(10):1072–3.

Index

Note: Page numbers of article titles are in **boldface** type.

Clin Liver Dis 13 (2009) 503–509
doi:10.1016/S1089-3261(09)00047-6

N

O

P

R

S

T

Printed and bound by CPI Group (UK) Ltd, Croydon, CR0 4YY
03/10/2024
01040464-0011